From Zero To Nurse

Excel in nursing school
Pass the NCLEX In 75
Secure your first job

SANDRAH NANZIRI, BSN RN

From Zero To Nurse
Sandrah Nanziri
First Edition
2019
Muttima Publishing

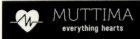

Editor: Shana Murph (Reedsy)
Cover Illustrator: Stewart Williams (Reedsy)
All rights reserved

Moral Rights
Sandrah Nanziri asserts the moral right to be identified as the author of this work.

External Content
Sandrah Nanziri has no responsibility for the persistence or accuracy of URLs for external or third-party Internet Websites referred to in this publication and does not guarantee that any content on such Websites is, or will remain, accurate or appropriate.

Designations
Designations used by companies to distinguish their products are often claimed as trademarks. All brand names and product names used in this book and on its cover are trade names, service marks, trademarks, and registered trademarks of their respective owners. The publishers and the book are not associated with any product or vendor mentioned in this book. None of the companies referenced within the book have endorsed the book.

In the loving memory of Emmanuel Kaasa Bajjabayira

#ForeverBaj

You will always be in our hearts

Dedication

To my family: This book is dedicated to each one of you. Thank you for bearing with me, believing in me, and supporting all my endeavors.

To my parents: Mr. Kaasa Charles and Mrs. Resty Tuta Nabukeera Lubega. I thank you both for taking me to the best schools and building a solid foundation for me. I am a result of academic discipline. I recall being sent home from school because my school dues were not paid on time but there was never a time you gave up on me. Mom, God bless your soul, you would encourage me to go the next day knowing I would be sent home again. You would say, "at least you won't miss everything". Thank you, mom, for being relentless when it came to my education. You always wanted the absolute best for us.

To all my siblings: I hope to inspire you to achieve more than the limits that are set for you. The sky is not the limit. It is only the beginning of what you are capable of. When you reach, opportunities will avail themselves to you. So, reach. I have walked the same road. "Everything will be okay," I want you to succeed.

To my friends: I promise to walk this path with you. I hope this is enough of a guide and much more.

Acknowledgements

Getting into nursing school, staying in school, and succeeding can be a challenge. My hope is that this book not only simplifies the process but also magnifies the gruesome process, so you are better equipped to navigate the program. For the students that approached me every day and asked how to best navigate the program and succeed, I have you to thank for helping me pen this book.

I also would like to extend gratitude to my fellow nurses that agreed to provide insight about the situations I never experienced. Thank you, Stephanie Rosario BSN RN, Nassiwa Kayondo BSN RN, Kelly Loretta BSN RN, Thatiana Jeune BSN RN, Diane Zatolokin BSN RN, and Mikayla Murphy BSN RN. Your insight will enlighten other nurses. Thank you!

To my professors and clinical instructors at Regis College, you are all wonderful. Thank you for believing in me and for answering my never-ending questions. You all functioned like a fine-tuned machine that churned out the most knowledgeable students, now nurses. I will forever be indebted to the world-class education Regis College offered. The loans incurred were worth it. Rose O my nursing preceptor and friend, thank you for being a mirror of what nursing is and should be.

To my first editor Beatrice Ada, your skills are impeccable. Thank you for perfecting this piece. To my second editor, Shana Murph, your knowledge of nursing enriched this text. Thank you for polishing this text and enabling me to deliver the message I intended to. I am grateful.

Table of Contents

Introduction

How did I get here? Why this book? Well, Zero to Nurse is something I wish I had when I was in nursing school—a guide, a detour when necessary, encouragement and reassurance that all is well that ends well. During my school years, I was approached by a lot of people, friends, family, and students who wanted to know how to navigate certain areas in nursing school. I pride myself in thinking I did well, but it would have been easier if I had this book.

A wise person once said, *"Smart people learn from their own mistakes, and a wise person learns from other peoples' mistakes."* In this book, I talk a lot about what I should have done differently and how I achieved success. This will not only help you avoid making mistakes, but it also cuts your preparation in half, therefore, saving you time.

This book is for every nursing student hopeful. I address nursing across the continuum—from interest, to learning, and all the way through to NCLEX testing, job searches and settling into your first year.

Who needs more books when nursing students are already assigned various books they are required to read? You do. You need this book, because this book is different. I promise you that. The average nursing text has anywhere from 400 to 1000 pages. I will teach you how to make appropriate use of your text without reading all 1000 pages, and how to pull out the need to know and the good to know.

In a way, I think the books assigned to us in nursing school prepare us for the real world. One day, when you become a nurse, you will receive nursing report on a patient assignment. You will get lots of information, some useful and some not so useful. When you do, you will have to prioritize the information into these two categories; the "need to know" and the "good to know." This practice starts before you even become a nurse. It starts in nursing school. From Zero to Nurse will address all these areas.

Nursing is a noble profession, one that relies heavily on evidence-based research. As you go through this book, you will find that I have used a lot of resources to support my experiences. For more information, go to the reference section of this book to further understand the content.

I love nursing. I loved learning, and here is what I learned in nursing school and my first year of practice. Nursing is a calling. If you have purchased this book, you my friend, have been called.

Sandrah Nanziri, BSN, RN

Prologue

W hat qualifies me to author a book about nursing? When I told someone, I was authoring a book, she asked me this question.

"What qualifies you to write a book about nursing?"

I am no writer. Always a reader, just never a writer. My idea of a writer is someone with writing prowess such as, Ernest Hemmingway, Charles Dickens, Chinua Achebe, etc. I just never imagined that I would author a book someday. The thing with writing is that you are called to tell a story and you never stop until it is heard.

I moved to the United States in January of 2010. I enrolled in a community college in 2012 to obtain an associate degree in nursing after having worked as a certified nurse assistant for a year. I then transferred to a four-year school in 2013 and graduated with honors in 2017. I was licensed to practice the same year after passing the NCLEX in 75 questions. These timelines are important to me because they represent years of hard work, perseverance, and success.

People around me at the time, discouraged me from pursuing nursing school. Some said, "I was not smart enough for the school system in the US," and that "I could not possibly pass the NCLEX on the first try because so many failed." They told me, "I would never be able to find a job in an acute hospital or work in the ICU." *From Zero to Nurse* is more than a guide for student nurses, it is a tale of what you can do if you work hard and believe in yourself.

I was compelled to write because I needed to create a resource for my siblings in nursing school. I found that during nursing school, I had a lot of questions and not so many answers. Students, aspiring nurses, and new nurses approached me and asked me if I could give them more information about different aspects of nursing school and if I could give them tips on obtaining a job. Authoring a book is my way of ensuring that someone else will have the resources to excel in the program and beyond. This is my way of paying it forward.

In my final year of nursing school, I started to write. To answer the question, "What qualifies me to a write a book about nursing?" I will say it is my experiences coupled with the triumphs, despite adversities, that qualify me to guide another nursing school hopeful, student, and novice nurse. I authored this book for you.

CHAPTER 1

My Nursing School Journey

I moved to the United States in 2010, and I come from quite a large family. A family of twelve, with four siblings currently in nursing school. My family and I lived in Ashland Massachusetts with an aunt for a while. Growing up, I loved science. Body systems (biology) and chemistry were my favorites. I always thought I would be a doctor because in Uganda, if you excel at sciences, you are more likely to become a doctor. Now that I am more exposed, I believe that I had limited nursing influences. Uganda (my country of origin) a former British colony mirrors the nursing system in Great Britain. Nurses to date wear dresses. I cannot imagine running to a code in a dress!

I had plans to go to medical school when I moved. Upon researching the requirements, funding and everything involved, I found the expenses and the time it would take to complete medical school overwhelming. In the meantime, I was exposed to the wonderful field of nursing. I had several doctors' appointments in my first year in the United States. I admired the nurses that treated me during this time. More than doctors, I interacted with nurses. Their knowledge level, compassion and care changed my views on nursing. I recall being amazed at how skillful one of the nurses was during a physical assessment. She was personable, wanted to know who I was and what I wanted to do. I spoke to her briefly about the medical field and she said, "Well, you are not too far from what you really want." This experience also reminds me of the importance of having a mentor or someone you can look up to. I knew of nursing, I just had minimal influences. I have a distant aunt, Sister Florence (May her soul RIP) who practiced as a nurse at a prominent hospital in Uganda. Her demeanor was very gentle, almost angelic, and she wore a dress to work. I can imagine she was a great nurse. I just never fancied dresses for work and never really spoke to her about her work duties. I regret that I never did. I presume she would have been an awesome mentor and influence.

I choose to pursue an education in nursing for so many reasons, including wanting to wear pants to work. Both fields (nursing and medicine) are rewarding, and I have not regretted my choice since. Nursing is such a gratifying field.

I enrolled at Massachusetts Bay Community College and started taking my nursing prerequisites with a plan to enroll in the Associates Degree Nursing Program. I never researched anything. I really relied on advice from relatives and friends. I wasted a lot of time and resources. I can tell you now that I regret having not pursued a four-year education immediately.

I listened to a lot of criticism from people that had no idea what I was capable of. Some people told me four-year colleges were hard and are structured for smart students. Ha-ha! Now that was funny. I knew I was very capable of excelling at a four-year college. The thoughts of others should never influence how you think of oneself.

A lot of people also told me I could not afford a four-year school; therefore, I should quit it all together. Well, that was partly true. I do not fault anyone for offering advice based on what they are exposed to. During this time, my mother was my rock. She repeatedly told me to remember who I was and that she knew I would find a way.

I transferred to Regis College from Massachusetts Bay Community College after taking most of my prerequisites. While transferring, some of the classes I had taken at the Community College did not transfer over (Again, a complete waste of time and resources). If you are thinking of going this route, that is, taking your pre-requisites at a community college before transferring to a four year school, I recommend that you visit the four-year school you have in mind and obtain the most recent nursing curriculum before you spend money and time on classes that will most likely not get transferred. Every school has requirements. When you visit potential schools, ask for a copy of the curriculum and only take classes that are transferable. It is also beneficial to meet with an advisor at a four-year school regularly to make sure you are on the right track.

On completing the credits that are most likely to transfer, waste no time. TRANSFER! I say so because I know of people that have taken breaks and never went back because life happened. Guess what, life is always going to happen, and it is never going to stop happening. Get in, stay in and you will figure things out. Even when life happens, you will find a way.

I would say taking classes at a community college is very flexible and it prepares you for the program. For a student like myself, one that had not been through the school system in the United States, community college prepared me for the demands of a four-year school.

When I was at the community college, I was able to work mornings and go to classes at night. Something that worked for me at the time. I also was able to take otherwise intense classes at a manageable pace. I took Anatomy and Physiology 1 and 2 at a community college. These classes, especially classes such as Anatomy and Physiology will prepare you for a four-year school. The content is the same. Taking these classes at a community college will also help you determine if pursuing a nursing education is for you. If you are still undecided about nursing school, you can enroll in a few nursing courses at a community college to test the waters. I have been asked whether the option of taking classes at a community college saves money. In my opinion, it is almost the same especially when you have a plan to transfer. You can save a few dollars because the cost per credit can be significantly less.

What to do After You have Transferred

So, you have transferred, or you are a first-year student with an interest in nursing. What is next? Being intentional and planning ahead of time makes for a good nursing student. At this point, you will be assigned an advisor. This advisor is your "nursing god." Listen to them, take their advice, and have an eagerness to learn (they can sense that), then they will do whatever it takes to make you successful in school and beyond. Before you meet with your advisor, prepare ahead of time. I recall my first meeting with my advisor. I totally blew it! I was not prepared to ask the most important questions. My advisor at the time said, "I doubt you will be successful in this program. You are ill prepared compared to your colleagues." The same advisor also said, "Since English is your second language, you will have to sign up for extra help". She totally ignored the fact that my GPA was greater than 3.6. I was expected to fail right from the start. This sent an action wave down my spine. At first, I was upset, then I planned to prove my worth for this intense program.

The best way to prepare for an advisor meeting is to write your questions on a piece of paper prior to the meeting. Again, this is a skill you will need to practice, the more you practice, the more second nature it becomes. Prepare before you meet with advisors and patients. It structures the meeting, and you get the most out of all your encounters. Some important questions to ask and remember are:

- How many classes do I need before I can be considered for entry into the program?

- What are the minimum GPA requirements?

- How many times can I retake a course before failing out of the program? (This question is important. It will help you to always strive for excellence)

- If possible, ask to look at the nursing curriculum. Know what is expected.

- Ask about all the resources available on and off campus.

- Ask advisors about classes (classes such as pathophysiology and pharmacology) that nursing students find challenging and gather material so you can tackle these classes.

- Ask how you are assigned classes and clinical rotations? If you can self-schedule nursing classes, or how soon one can sign up. When your nursing sign-up schedule opens, be vigilant. Find out which instructors will help you succeed. Ask senior nursing students' which instructors are in tune with their student population. You can also use **ratemyproffessors.com.**

Also, if you should find yourself in a position where the advisor-student nurse relationship is not working, seek a change through the right channels. Never, I repeat NEVER burn bridges and/or relationships in nursing; it is a small world. Believe me.

Schools are different. So, it is important to know the stipulations. Once you have enrolled, obtain a copy of the nursing curriculum, and check off completed requirements as you go. Be your own advocate. If possible, acquire a copy of your graduating class's required courses. Before you take or sign up for a class, MAKE SURE THE CLASS IS WITHIN THE REQUIREMENTS. Sometimes advisors are overwhelmed by the student body they serve, and yes, they can make mistakes. It is okay to consult with your classmates, just do not approach advisors with the "how come so and so is not taking this class?" Always make sure to solicit information from the right sources (this is particularly important). Nursing students are some of the most anxious individuals I ever have come across. They panic over ANYTHING. Every one of them has a different answer to a comparable situation. Make sure your information is right.

You will be assigned to an academic advisor. Take down their email and contact information and store it someplace. This is your go-to-person for everything academic in nature. Email them, respectfully. Notice I said, respectfully. I cannot stress the importance of being respectful. While in nursing school, we are consumers of education. The adage "the customer is the boss" barely applies. This profession is a multidisciplinary profession, and it is important that you begin to practice respect along with professionalism. Yes, you are paying a lot, so will your clients and/or patients. Be professional and respectful. Working with multiple individuals requires respect. You will notice that students who are respectful perform better and instructors and faculty are more inclined to assist them.

Ideally, you will have your class schedule before the commencement of the semester. Plan wisely. One thing that stresses students out, is the failure to harmonize work, school, and social life schedules. Plan to work when you are not in school. I scheduled my work on weekends even though I hated working every weekend. During weekdays, I focused on school and school alone. With a schedule like mine, there's hardly time for a social life. Anything can be put on hold. The amount of dedication will surely pay off. It did for me.

You should allocate 1-3 hours a day to relieve stress, and then you can plan social activities. Build a self-care routine to help you combat stress in nursing school. Remember, the habits you build while in nursing school, are likely to sustain you in a professional role. Your winter and summer breaks are times to be very selfish with your time and do everything you missed doing while in school. This practice will enable you to start every semester rejuvenated and content. Remember, nursing school is temporary, you can survive a few years of deprivation. No one has died from that.

Write down all your assignment deadlines and back date the deadline by a week. If your assignment is due on March 5th, mark the due date as February 26th. When you check your due deadlines, you will know that you have a week left to complete the assignment. This habit will help you stay ahead. With the technology these days, I am sure you can even set alarm reminders a week before assignments are due. This helps you plan better and hand in assignments that are well thought of. To succeed in this program, you must take every assignment seriously. Getting your assignments done effectively helps you learn much more from the assignment.

You know what they say, experience is the best teacher. Most of the things I mention in this book are things that I have done that guaranteed my success. However, there are a few things that I could have done differently and much better. I will mention those too, so you know what not to do.

I would also want every one of you that has been criticized, advised wrongly, discouraged, and overlooked to know that you can excel. My capabilities have been measured based on the color of my skin and having an accent, background and much more. But nothing I endured broke me down or changed my views about nursing as a profession. If anything, these experiences have taught me to reach out to those that have been subjected to the same judgments and encourage them to focus on what matters.

Every single day, you define who you are, what you stand for and what you will become. If someone ever told you, you are incapable of being a nurse, I say to you; YOU ARE CAPABLE! No one knows you as well as you know yourself. When you push forward, you break barriers. I came across an interesting concept called grit that defined my drive-in nursing school and in life. Grit explains why some people regardless of lack of talent and/or capabilities are successful.

GRIT

I personally think that the most successful students are the gritty ones. Having the right attitude is your lifeline in nursing school. Some days will knock you down more than others. But the rise after the fall, the perseverance and resilience is what will get you through. In one word, you have "GRIT."

Why grit? I love watching TED talks in my free time and I play them when I am driving, while I am on the train and when I need some inspiration. Those speakers are very smart people, and because of the time constraints, they get straight to the point.

One day I searched the term perseverance because at that time, I was drained. My search led me to Angela Lee's Duckworth TED talk about grit. See I am a gritty individual, but I have never come across a word that defines my drive and passion until the day I listened to her talk.

According to Angela, "grit is the belief in the achievement of long-term goals that drives one to do whatever is possible to succeed." The long-term goal in your case is becoming an RN.

Grit is an essential characteristic that every nursing student should have. The truth is that nursing school is hard. I do however think that a student that has made up their mind up to succeed and do whatever is necessary will triumph.

I have witnessed not so smart students perform incredibly well and therefore become successful in the program. These students do whatever is necessary to succeed. They study, make use of resources, and go the extra mile. All these habits are necessary for you to do well in nursing school.

Just as the fingers on your hand are unequal, so are we as individuals. Some individuals will succeed without working excessively hard. These are your outliers, and that makes up for less than five percent of the aspiring nursing students' population. The rest of us must do the work. A lot of nurses you meet will tell you nursing school was tough, but everything was worth it.

Prior to the start of the semester, that is before entry into the nursing program, I took a standardized national ATI test which determines one's ability to succeed in the program. I was placed below the national average for math and English and above the national average for science. When you look at my current ATI results after entry into the program and compare them to students that had a higher entry level, I am above the average national level in all subjects. Because I am a gritty individual, I never let that "standardized testing tool" determine how well I would do in the program. My first nursing school advisor even recommended that I need remedial classes because English is a second language. I remember tearfully telling her that I can do it and will do it and I did not need remedial classes. I went ahead to place myself at an advantage in the end.

Failure is not a permanent condition, especially in nursing school but in life as well. What you do after you fail is what determines how you turn out.

Never let a test score lower your self-expectations. Continue to believe in yourself and do what it takes. You are going to come across various obstacles, but your self-belief is what is going to get you ahead.

Like many, my first nursing exam score was a shock—I got a 78.5%. The pass grade was 80%. Having been an A student prior to this score, I was deeply disappointed. I learned very quickly that nursing school examinations are different. The multiple- choice tests usually have two correct options; the answer is the best of the two choices.

This did not make sense in the beginning, and I was frustrated but instead of lingering on the score, I went back to the drawing board. With the help of faculty, I reevaluated the way I studied. I had to change the way I compartmentalized information. I re-assessed myself, determined that I had to change my learning needs and then use different resources.

By the third test, I had figured things out and was scoring high 90s on tests. I finally understood why it is important to follow the nursing process while answering questions. Deep down I knew that I could do better, and I never let one bad score determine my future in nursing school. I wanted to be a nurse, and this meant doing everything I could, to make it in the program. That is grit.

You usually have at least four exams in a semester, so never ruminate failure because it impedes your ability to move forward. Take what you are handed and do something about it.

A gritty student will be driven by their passion and drive. Passion and drive awaken one's perseverance. Like the nursing process, I implore students to assess their ability to make it through the program. I also have used the nursing process throughout this book to reinforce the concept.

Grit Assessment Tool

- How gritty are you?
- Write down the reasons you are pursuing this program.
- After you have sieved through the reasons, pick your top three. Those three reasons should reawaken your drive when you fall short.
- Write them down on a piece of cardboard and place them in a room you use every day. If you face a challenge, go back to those reasons, and reevaluate what you need to do to overcome the challenge. Let these reasons inspire you.

I am not the best writer, and I do not take pride in being a strong writer but here I am writing. How? I have this image in my head of the cover of this book even before completion. This image implores me to take time out of every day to write a few thousand words. There are days that my writing runs exceedingly low. It is at these times that I return to the start. Every time I visualize the book cover, my drive is reawakened, I suddenly have something to write about. With nursing school, you can envision your day of graduation, cap, gown, and tassel in hand or adding credentials to your name. Use that to inspire you when you are challenged.

I have heard too many inspiring tales of perseverance through nursing school. Single mothers that walked across the stage to receive their diplomas, students that failed out before excelling, immigrant students that did not speak any English the first day of class only to pass with excellence at the end, students that failed out of nursing programs excelling when they tried at other colleges… The motivation and passion therein, the tears, the burdens and everything that could have torn them apart and failed them in the process only molded them into something much stronger.

To tell you the truth, anything is possible if you believe in your long-term goals. The belief in oneself will mask the arduous work, and instead of detesting nursing school, you will love it, and you will work hard unknowingly. Always remember that pressure builds diamonds, and all of this is temporary. I have met too many nurses that say it is all worth it in the very end, and there is no reason not to believe them. There will always be light at the end of the tunnel.

A colleague of mine, a licensed practical nurse, failed out of a registered nurse program. She now has signed up for classes in another

RN program. I could tell that this time she was going to be successful because she mentioned that she is ready to do whatever it takes.

Many times, it is not about how brilliant one is, it is the resilience that enables mediocre students to be remarkably successful in these programs. A past failure should never detour you from your dreams.

In conclusion, grit is very necessary. On a scale of one to ten, one being no grit and ten being very gritty, how gritty are you? If you find that you have not made up your mind about nursing school but are interested, I implore you to find inspiration, drive, and determination first.

Your long-term goals will be the ones to get you up in the wee hours of the night to review material. They will be the same ones to fill you up when your drive runs empty. Determine how gritty you are about nursing school before you start.

For the students that have failed out of the program. You still have a chance especially if this is what you really want. There are lots of nursing schools. Only your grit will get you through this process. How bad do you want it and how willing are you to get up and try again? Grit got me through nursing school, NCLEX testing and then securing a job. I believed I could, every step of the way. Therefore, it is important to know right from the start why you are pursuing nursing and assess oneself fully. In the next chapter, we review self-assessment. Assessment is the initial step in the nursing process. Start off your nursing journey the right way.

CHAPTER 2

Nursing, Self-Assessment and Self-Care

And so, it begins...

Are you thinking about attending nursing school? Do you want to learn how to navigate the process and find out how to start? Everything in life begins with a goal. First, there is a goal. Then, there is a plan and then the implementation of said plan. But before all of that, there is the heart. You must have what it takes to become a nurse. You must have heard the notion that nursing is the work of the heart. It takes passion, compassion, a willingness to serve others and impact lives.

It is essential to know why you want to pursue nursing. Why do you want to be a nurse? This is the most important question you will have to ask yourself before commencing this journey. So, think clearly, be articulate, and be honest with yourself.

Self-Assessment

Compassion and passion are a huge component of nursing. What are your reasons for seeking out this career? This is what draws the line between a good nurse and a not so good nurse. Are you one to care deeply for others? Who are you as a person? Are you fair in the decisions you make? Are you judgmental? All these questions are things you should take time to think about. Remember, honesty is the best policy. Assess your prejudices. Being aware of them is a step closer to changing these beliefs.

Yes, compassion can be learned and so can many other characteristics. I have witnessed several excellent students that barely care about the art of nursing. These students usually encompass the science in nursing. They understand the concepts, and they are extremely brilliant, but they lack the humanity component. They lack the ability to connect with the people they serve but will be able to critically think through any disease process. Nursing cannot weed these types of students out because they are excellent students. The expectation is that they will grow into it. Some do, some never do. I am sure many of you have come across similar characters. I believe nursing is both an art and a science.

I know of one very brilliant new nurse who will walk into a patient's room, give medications utilizing all the 7 rights of medication administration, perform an exceptional head to toe assessment, and walk out without engaging the patient. This individual is always on time and completes all their nursing assignments and stated duties.

Then there's another individual that walks into the rooms of patients, introduces him/herself; asks to open the blinds so she can let more light into the room; asks patients if they had a good night's sleep; asks how they like to take their pills and what they would like to take their pills with; takes out a dirty tray and before walking out the room, he/she asks patients if they would need something upon return. This individual then returns to the room with patient medication. She lets patients know what medications they are taking and what side effects to report and/or expect (even though the patient has heard them a thousand times). Then, as he/she administers the medication, he/she also asks if the patient has any concerns or questions, performs an assessment while engaging the patient and then proceeds to let the patient know what to expect during the day. Before the nurse walks out, she proceeds to ask if there is anything else the patient needs.

Having read those two examples? Which of those two nurses would you like to be? This is the difference between a good nurse and a not so good nurse. I have worked with both kinds, and I can assure you, no matter the work load, a good nurse always finds a way to engage with his or her patients on a different level. I have had nurses give report and say the patient is difficult and then that same patient ends up relating to the oncoming nurse and builds a therapeutic relationship with him/her. I gave this example to encourage you to evaluate why you are choosing nursing. Because there is more to nursing. Nursing is both a science and an art. The two should synchronize to birth a great nurse. I want you to investigate what nursing is and what nursing is not.

Nursing is also a profession defined by relationships. I think building relationships is an art. To do our job, we rely on relationships to work. We build relationships with our patients (most important), with co-workers (equally important), with the organizations we work with, and with the systems we practice in and much more. Many nurses will tell you that what we are doing is customer care in the health field. The difference is, our customers are patients. If you do not like working with people, you will have a rude awakening. You need to love working with people.

These are some of the things you should think about before entering this profession. There is a lot more to this subject than I can relay. If you are not sure about entering the profession, I would advise you to work in a health-related field first. Observe nurses at work and decide if you like what they do before making the decision. In otherwise, make an informed decision to pursue nursing.

There is also a popular misconception about pay. Some people have pursued this profession for job security. Please remember that at the end of the day, you are working with human beings at their worst. These people are relying on you to meet their needs and relieve their pain. It is only fair that you do your absolute best. There is no test for compassion. However, your conscious, if you have one, will hold you accountable. Please choose this profession for the right reasons. There are arguments about finding your nursing niche. A lot of times people are better nurses when they work with the populations they can relate with or are compassionate about. If that is the case, work with a population that brings the best out of you.

What do you aspire to be?

What do you hope to achieve from nursing? In fact, where do you hope to practice? What kind of nursing are you interested in? In the beginning, you will find out that you want to be a certain kind of nurse. This decision can change or remain the same with experience. The more you are exposed to the plethora of options, the harder the decision becomes for some student nurses.

I wanted to be a pediatric nurse in the beginning. I had no doubt that I wanted to work with kids. See, I have eleven siblings. How hard can that be? Been there, done that. Right? At least that is what I thought. Two years later, I realized that I am a fast-paced learner and that I love thinking things through. I am also very inquisitive and seem to enjoy delving deeper into things. I am always looking out for change, following trends to know when things are not right and voila! I realized that I am best fit for trauma or intensive care. I did not figure this out overnight.

It was a series of classes, clinical rotations, and peer input. My peers were usually annoyed by my need to understand complex information. Your best fit as a nurse must align with who you are as an individual. This is not too far from who I am as an individual.

This decision was confirmed during my senior practicum on an intensive cardiac unit. I loved it! I often said, this is so me. I have been told that the clinical you enjoyed the most is your best fit. This is true for most people, but not everyone so, take your time. Write your hopes down, travel through the journey and you shall soon arrive at your calling. As a nursing student, go through all experiences with an open mind, if you love it, pursue it. Experience is the best teacher.

Be honest with yourself, assessing oneself is key. The better you get at knowing who you are and what you want, the easier it will be for you to rightfully place yourself. You will learn why it is so important to be attentive to yourself. So, start now. Construct a vision board and map your way to the end goal that is nursing. Using affirmation, the title of the vision board should be the proposed year of graduation. If you graduate in 2019, the vision board title should be_____BSN, RN 2019, or RN 2019. By printing your legal name and future title, you have manifested this into your future and the universe will then work with you to make your dreams come true.

Nursing Vision Board Ideas

Who are you?

Print your name and title with the year of graduation.

What defines you?

What do you enjoy doing? What are your favorite hobbies? It is important to know who we are and what we love as individuals. Remember, the things you love can be incorporated into nursing because you are working with people. I know of nurses that are fitness gurus that have gone on to become healthy living advocates, and nurses that love skin care that are now aesthetic nurses. I once met a Reiki nurse once that found her calling after following her path of interest. She now travels to acute care hospitals, rehabilitations, and performs Reiki.

I personally love clothes and dressing up was always a passion of mine. I recently opened an online nurse shop making unique ethnic print scrub tops. Knowing who you are as a person will help channel you into the type of nursing you want to do.

I mentioned listing your hobbies because I also want you to get in the habit of taking care of oneself early in your career.

A lot of times, your hobbies are ways you can self-care. Listing these hobbies will be a reminder to continue to do these things while in nursing school and beyond. Nursing is not a bed of roses. There is a lot of stress that comes with the job and nursing school. When you continue to care for yourself, you will never run low. You will also be a better caregiver. Let us take a closer look at caring for yourself.

Self-Care

You are looking into joining a profession that is centered on taking care of others. Do you realize how draining that is? Yes, you are passionate about taking care of others but who is taking care of you? The only way you can effectively take care of others is by taking better care of yourself.

Nurses have exited the profession prematurely because of the requirements of bedside nursing. As a new nurse, I cannot speak to those that have years of practice behind them. What I can speak on is having a system in place to take care of yourself. *Learning how to perform self-care starts in nursing school. The habits you build in nursing school can potentially follow you into the profession.*

Self-care begins with a thorough assessment of self. Identify stressors and what ways you have utilized in the past to cope under pressure. I am introducing self-care early because it is important to cultivate a system right from the very beginning.

While researching the topic itself, I found that a lot of nurses utilize their hobbies as a means of self-care, performing activities such as, hiking, eating healthy, workouts, travel, skin care, massages, spending quality time with loved ones, etc. Whatever that activity is, make sure it is relieving stress. Sometimes you outgrow previously learned coping skills/methods. The good news is that you can always learn new ways to perform self-care.

Do you have a self-care method in place? If not, let us go over a few key areas in finding a self-care method;

- List your hobbies. Do you feel fulfilled and nourished after partaking in your hobbies? Say one loves drawing. Does the act of drawing help you organize your thoughts and thereby become less stressed about day-to-day life?

- Are the existent self-care methods maladaptive? That is, not helping relive stress and anxiety. Conduct a self-assessment and start all over.

- Do you know of nurses that have crafted self-care methods that are effective? I started a Self-Care for Nurses series on my blog to encourage other nurses to share their self-care activities. This forum is a means for nurses to learn from one another and inspire others to take care of themselves. To participate or learn about what other nurses are doing, follow **@nurseyscrubs on Instagram** and tell us how you practice self-care so we can share with other nurses and learn from each other.

- Take time out of your day to practice self-care. Dedicate that time to fulfilling oneself (body, mind, and soul). I have found that defining the day, time, and activities one will partake in is a way of being accountable to self. I call these days, my **Do Not Disturb (DND)** days. My perfect self-care day involves going to the gym, getting a full body massage, and then taking a scrub bath. I also light lavender candles in the bathroom prior to showers. Lavender is known for its ability to aide in relaxation.

- While choosing a self-care activity, remember that health encompasses body, mind, and soul. Your mental health is equally important. How do you know that you are mentally drained? What activities can help restore your mental health balance? Visiting a trained professional, practicing mindfulness, and checking in occasionally are some of the ways one can take care of themselves mentally.

Again, to get better at this, one must commit to the idea of living a fulfilling life. Our job as nurses is rewarding but do not let the demands of the workplace get you to a point where you are leaving the profession all together because of compassion fatigue. As a new nurse, be firm in the need to care for oneself. Make a commitment to ALWAYS care for self-first. Nursing students usually build their self-care habits in nursing school. Make sure the habits you are building are sustainable over time and most importantly, are effective in relieving anxiety and stress. Self-care is the best care.

YOU HAVE WHAT IT TAKES, START TODAY.

CHAPTER 3

Finances and Cutting Expenses

N ursing school is expensive. That is the truth. That in no way should discourage you from pursuing the process. First, you need to assess your individual financial situation. Then, figure out how you are going to pay for it. Some students transfer from high school with scholarships. That is great. Others have financial support from parents and relatives. That is ideal as well. I went to school with someone whose education was fully funded by a grandparent. If you have neither, worry less. I will guide you the best way I can. I know that every problem has a solution.

Assessing One's Financial Readiness and Status

Are you paying for school? If so, this is a very crucial area to assess prior to enrolling in nursing school. Unfortunately, it is one of the key factors that determine how successful you will be. Students from poor backgrounds have dropped out of Baccalaureate programs because they cannot afford to pay for tuition and other expenses that are a part of the nursing program. Primarily, the books are expensive. There were some semesters that required no less than $300 in book purchases per semester. These books were also mandatory and frequently used in course work. One could not afford to do without them. Refer to the section "Nursing School Books" to learn how you can cut back on book expenses.

Do you know how much are you are able to pay for nursing school? You must know the answer to this question before enrolling. Community colleges will cost you at least $150 to $250 a credit, and private schools range from $1000-$1500 a credit. The only advantage of going to private schools is the smaller class size and overall attention to detail. Otherwise, a great nurse is great nurse. It does not matter what school the nurse attended.

Knowing your expenses ahead of time will prepare you for the tougher decisions such as why your credit score is very crucial in attaining loans, and the importance of having a cosigner, financial aid, and student loans. If someone is paying for your education, consider that a blessing because without them, the struggle is very real.

Learn about Credit, Credit Scores, and Co-Signers

What about credit scores? We all have heard the saying that "America runs on Dunkin'." Well, I think America runs on credit. The better your credit, the easier it is to access anything. Your life is ten times harder with a low credit. Good credit is a necessity even in nursing school.

A good credit score will allow you to take out student loans to finance your own education. This message is for students that are taking a front row seat in paying for their education. There is no bank, credit bureau or student loaning company that will offer a loan to someone with low or poor credit. I moved to this country a few years ago, and I wish that I had taken a class on credit to better understand how to build and sustain good credit. These are things I did not contemplate. But lesson learned. If you have zero knowledge about credit, take a class or consult an expert and learn the ins and outs of building and sustaining credit. I personally feel that anyone that was not raised in America needs to undergo some form credit education.

Until very recently, I never realized how important it was to have an excellent credit score. Coming from a different country, credit was not an understood concept. This is one of the things that will serve you for life, and I would highly recommend that you become aware of your credit scores and maintain good scores. Banks offer up to $75,000 in student loans with great interest rates for students with good credit and you might not need a co-signer for loans.

I would also advise that if one is capable, pay the interest rates of your student loans while in school and upon graduation, consolidate all your student loans. This will enable you to make reasonable payments toward your loans.

If you lack good credit, having a cosigner with a strong credit score is an added advantage. If you are not able to meet the requirements to get student loans, you will be asked to provide a co-signer who is just as responsible for the loan as you are. This part is important. Do not overlook it. Many of the students I went to school with had their parents co-signing their loans with the expectation that upon graduation, they will be able to pay the loans.

Figuring out Financial Aid

Understanding financial aid is so vital. There are a couple of key features to know such as meeting application deadlines, promissory notes, and exit cancelling to mention but a few. Solicit information from credible sources. To understand the way financial aid works, how much you owe, and how to complete the paperwork, you will need to contact the financial aid office. A good rule of thumb is to prepare for this meeting ahead of time and be prepared to ask as many questions as you see fit. These offices are there to assist you and you would rather acquire information from them than other secondary sources.

Paying for School While in School

A have a few nurse friends that attended community college and graduated with no debt to their names. One of them worked two jobs, studied on the job, and never had any free time. You must have excellent time management and academic skills to succeed while

35

doing this. This individual also worked twice as hard in the summer and saved up for the rainy days while in school. She had five months payments saved for all the bills she had (car note, rent, gas, phone, and food). There were no surprises.

Yes, this is ideal, but the stress related to pursing an education without a loan can be overwhelming. You want to make it through this rigorous program and such a commitment will not only burden you but also affect your academic life. As a nursing student, you should be able to have a balance between work and school. If you commit to paying for school while in school, you will work more and have less time to study.

Despite how difficult it is, working and paying for school while in school is possible, especially if it is a low-cost community college. You can save enough to pay for the credits you are taking per semester and you will graduate debt free.

A lot of these students that have graduated without loans are older, adult scholars, if I may. These students sacrificed a lot to make ends meet. If you have this sort of financial discipline, this is a route you can take.

I on the other hand went to a private school. Despite the scholarships and financial aid, I found that I always had a school balance at the end of the school year. In my final year, I ran out of financial aid. Yes, there is a limit. When you first enroll, find out how much you must spend in financial aid and plan accordingly.

I remember visiting the financial aid office to discuss the best way to move forward. The advisor recommended that I take time off from school to work and save up for school. This is something I am strongly against. I have seen people take time off and never return to school because life happened. Yes, some people return, but a lot of them do not, and I did not want to be part of that statistic. That for me was not an option.

As an older student, I had less family financial support and relied solely on myself to meet all requirements. If you are older and wish to go to nursing school, I would say have a good amount of money saved up for rainy days before embarking on the journey. I strongly advise against taking breaks from school unless of course the reason is beyond your control. The nursing learning curve connects dots, and with every break, you stand a chance of falling off and you end up doing more work to get back on track.

I graduated with a school balance of $12,000 and a lot more in outside loans. This meant that I could not take my board exams until I cleared this balance. I tried several avenues, but I was unsuccessful in my quest. It is important to include this piece because I would like to prepare you well enough so that you can avoid an experience such as mine. Upon graduation, I did not receive my diploma or transcript, and this made me quite sad, but it was expected. I knew what I needed to do so I made plans to resolve the issue. This meant that I would be working full time and I would take the NCLEX exam much later than expected. I was ready to take the NCLEX the month after graduating but I was not able to do so because of financial reasons.

Another way to reduce the loan burden is to apply for scholarships ahead of time to cover tuition costs and books.

Nursing schools are expensive. Four-year schools to be exact. You need a plan, especially if like me, you have little to no financial support. Applying for financial aid way before the due date enables you to have room to fulfill other requirements that are requested after the application. Stay in close contact with the financial aid office and determine what scholarships are available on and off campus.

Applying for Scholarships

There are multiple scholarships online. Search the web, ask peers that are ahead of you and apply before they are due. Most scholarships have requirements due mid-May or the beginning of January. This is something I did not do until my senior year. Apply to as many scholarships as you can and keep your fingers crossed for consideration. Join nursing organizations to have access to their student scholarships.

Build respectable relationships with your professors, nursing colleagues, and clinical instructors. With scholarships, you will need a lot of letters of recommendation. So, having difficult relationships with your professional network will slow you down in this arena. Do not do it just for scholarships, get in the habit of being respectful because you must be and the profession you are entering requires you to always maintain respect.

Once you apply for a scholarship, write down the scholarship information, and monitor your email frequently for responses. Many students will tell you that they have been unsuccessful with attaining scholarships. There are multiple applicants, but you will never be lucky if you do not try. Once you have applied to various scholarships, you will know the tools you need, and the process will be easier than the first time. Some of the requirements scholarships always look for are; financial need from the financial office, letters of recommendation from faculty and work places, essays, and transcripts, affiliations to nursing organizations, desired outcomes such as working with a sustain population after graduation.

Searching for scholarships is an intense process of its own. These are things you can do while on school break. Remember to make copies of the letters of recommendations and save them. Also, maintain your grade point average as stated by the scholarship fund. You really do not want to lose your scholarship once you have gained one. Maintaining your GPA is possible and doable with the right amount of work.

For the students that work full and part-time in health institutions, visit the HR offices, and determine what reimbursements you are eligible for. If you have worked at the institution for some time, you should be eligible for school reimbursements among other things. Take everything you can get.

Financial constraints can be surpassed when we search for the resources that are available to us. Search the Internet for nursing organizations. Obtain the list online and look at individual organizations to determine if you possess the requirements, then apply. I would advise compiling a portfolio of frequently required scholarship requirements. That way, you are always prepared.

If you are interested in serving in the US Army. There are scholarship opportunities available whereby you will be deployed as an active duty officer upon graduation. Search health resources and services administration (HRSA) for available opportunities. The Nurse Corps Scholarship will require you to work in an area that is critically short of nurses upon graduation.

If you have the option of enrolling into a state school, you should consider that before attending private school. The thing about education is that it is an absolute sacrifice, and you are going to have to live below your means to succeed. Nursing is one of the fields where you will always have a job. If you must obtain loans, that is fine too. Worry about the loans after you graduate and even then, you are practically guaranteed to find work, which will enable you to pay off the loans.

Before you apply for loans, always exhaust the resources around you and borrow only what you need.

Nursing School Books

Another expense you will have during nursing school is books. Not only are the sizes of nursing books threatening, but they are also very costly. It does not help that you are never likely to use the same book and edition as the previous year. Having friends in high places is not helpful either in terms of using material from a year before. The editions or the whole text might be different. This I found unfair.

You also have the option of buying or renting from cheaper websites as opposed to campus book stores. Search the Web for available choices. I personally used Valore books, and I can confirm that it is awesome despite the ridiculously long shipping wait time. To counteract that, you can order books at least one month or two before school starts so that they are on time for the semester. I once purchased my books late and had to wait until the third week of school to have a text to refer to. Amazon is also a great resource. You can buy used books at a lower cost.

Make friends with students a semester ahead of you. You can even go as far as selecting the same instructors/professors and taking the same classes, that way, you are able to use texts from the previous class.

Libraries usually have texts on reserve. However, there are books you must purchase because they have links to on-line questions you can use to study from in your own time. Make sure to know all your resources and maximize them. I am so big on knowing your resources. It is like having a plan A, B, C and Z.

Cutting Expenses

You need to limit all your expenditures especially if you have minimal financial support. I drove an old car all through nursing school because I could not afford to pay an expensive car payment. I had a 2000 model in 2015 parked beside newer models. Yes, students in my school drove expensive cars. At first it bothered me, but then I redirected my energy to focusing on excelling in school. I had money to spend on other requirements because I was not making exorbitant car or insurance payments. My car insurance cost was $150 a month and I did not have a car note. I planned to cut costs by any means necessary.

The other thing I did was move back to my parent's house to avoid paying rent. In the beginning, I lived in a town twenty minutes from my school, but that cost me. Expenses such as groceries and other utilities strained my pockets and stressed me out. I made the decision to move back home and have extra money available when I needed it as opposed to having an empty account.

Commuting To School

I commuted through nursing school. I therefore can only speak for commuter students because I was one throughout my college life. Talking about my commuter experience, budgets and cutting costs may benefit a student that is looking to commute to school.

I lived in a Boston suburb, which was about 15.2 miles away from school. On a good day without traffic, it took me about half an hour to get to school. The routes were always backed up, so I gave myself an hour on most days. I found that I would still be late a lot of times, so I started to leave my house in the wee hours of the morning. On exam days, I left as early as 4:00 am.

Being a commuter student meant that I never saw my family for the most part because I was either on my way to school or on my way to work from school. When I left for the day, I had my work uniform parked. I was in and out of the house, and when I was there, I was sleeping and secluded in my room. In the beginning, my routine was cumbersome. Once I was accustomed to it, it was less cumbersome.

Being a commuter student is a challenge. If you can afford living at school, then live at school. You must plan; for transport, gas, car breakdowns, maintenance, and related expenses. You also must plan for meals as well. Because as you will find, school cafeterias are a rip-off. The food is unhealthy and expensive. In nursing school, you are living on a budget, so you must be smart with your money.

The best way to get around food expenses is to make home meals. I however found it hard to make home meals because I was exhausted most days and sometimes, I had to leave school and head straight to work. I barely had time. For a student with similar challenges, I would say that you must put aside money for food. The key to never lacking is to always make a budget and stick to it.

There will be times that even with a budget you will be deficient. My friend and I used to support each other by buying each other lunch or dinner that way we still had lunch when we needed to. Your support systems can come in handy with food expenses and everything related. One of my nursing colleagues also had weekly pre-parked frozen lunches from home and would share meals with her roommate.

Your schedule as a commuter student is a lot more complex than a student that lives at school. You will find that you cannot participate in many activities at school and will miss out on having a good college experience because you only make plans to be at school when you must be there and you must leave just when the college socials start. You will sit in awful traffic, and many times you will be tardy. It takes a lot of discipline to be punctual, pay related expenses, and stick to a budget, but I will say that it gets easier with time.

At the beginning of my commuter experience, I was late to every class. One day as I was reviewing my instructor's comments, I saw that she wrote that I was tardy 70% of the time. My grades were good. I just was never on time. That was the point at which I decided that I would no longer run late. I started leaving for school hours ahead of time to avoid traffic and surprises.

The other thing you can also do is try to become friends with someone who lives at school or find a family member that lives within the area. There will be days when these people come in handy. During exam days, I stayed over at a boyfriend's house. He lived 15 minutes away from campus. I could not afford to be late for tests, and I was able to arrive earlier to review my notes one last time before exams. Being late for exams is nerve wrecking and makes you very anxious. We all know how detrimental anxiety is during tests.

Snow days are a commuter's worst nightmare. Schools usually cancel on heavy snow days. But on the days, they do not cancel, you still must show up to class. As a nursing student, I tried not to miss any class unless of course, I had a good reason to. You will find that you miss a lot of content when you do not show up. Then, you are tasked with not only catching up, but also connecting the missing dots yourself. With the workload already placed on us, this is not ideal. Having a friend at school, a family member or friend that lives within the school vicinity will come handy on days like these.

The Unexpected

You would think that as a commuter student, investing in a good car would be a priority. It was however not the case on my end. Remember, in nursing school, the expenses are high, and the resources are insufficient. My car was too old and gave me trouble. A LOT. My friends even named her "Old Betsy" but hey, she got me through school and started me off in my professional life.

As I mentioned earlier, I tried to eliminate any expenses outside of school to cut down on stress. Despite Old Betsy's occasional breakdowns, we were fine up until we (myself and Old Betsy) were involved in a minor accident. Because I cut my expenses to minimal or none, my insurance coverage was a waste. It did not cover repairs. I had to put Old Betsy in a garage and cough up to $1200 in repairs. If you can afford it, invest in a new car, or drive a parent's car like most of my friends did.

With this unexpected turn in events, I still had to show up for my classes. Living 15.2 miles away from school did not help matters. Lucky enough, this happened in my very last semester, and I was only at school two days out of the week. My commuting involved walking to the bus stop, taking a train into Boston, and getting on the green line for about 50 minutes to a stop closest to school. I would then wait for the school shuttle to drop me off at school. This new development involved planning around the school shuttle schedule. I had to leave home at 5 am to be at school by 8:30 am. This went on for at least a month and a half. My friend would occasionally scoop me up from the train station, and I would ride with her to school and sometimes she would drop me off at the train stop on her way back home and vice versa.

I talk about this experience because in life we make plans, but things sometimes go wrong. It is wise to plan for events such as accidents, traffic, and car breakdowns. Always have a miscellaneous account set aside to cover costs should need be. In the summer time, make sure to work and save up for rainy days while in school. Being very disciplined with your income and expenditures is important.

I am sure some of the cons of commuting are eliminated for students that live on campus. I will say that I loved commuting and I am glad that I was able to make it through school. I went to a private school, and the expense of living at school is enormous. If given this option again, I would still commute.

Please be financially awakened by my experience. Knowing what to expect and planning is not only crucial in nursing school but in life as well. I always say the end justifies the means. A made it through school with a 2000 model (My dear Old Betsy) and I excelled while at it.

I want everyone to benefit from this book. Because I have no experience living on a school campus, I asked my colleagues, Kayondo Nassiwa, BSN RN and Thatiana Jeune BSN RN to give students that live on campus more insight about the pros and cons of living on campus.

Interview with Kayondo Nassiwa, BSN, RN about living on campus

1. Did living on campus ease nursing school? If yes, explain how.

I personally feel that living on campus did ease nursing school a bit. The reason as to why was the sense of community. There were many occasions that when I was overwhelmed during nursing school, I found support in fellow nursing students who also lived on campus.

I was able to see that I was not alone and that certain topics are easier for some than others.

2. In your opinion, is living on campus more favorable for a nursing student?

I believe that living on campus is more favorable. I also feel that it depends on the individual. Based on me, however, I thought it was more convenient living on campus because I could always meet up with professors and take advantage of opportunities that gave me extra learning time. I also think it is better because you create more of a sense of community being around your nursing student counterparts. It also gives you the opportunity to get involved in school programs that you might not want to drive from home for. I feel like being on campus kept me busy, but also made me more well-rounded as a person.

3. What challenges did you face as nursing student living on campus?

A big challenge that I faced was distraction. Just how I mentioned that being on campus can help you be more interested in participating in programs that the school has to offer, it can also cause you to not be as focused. As for me, a big problem for me was procrastination. Knowing that there were events going on when I had a test the same week was challenging. But it also helped me to perfect my time management skills and set my priorities.

4. How did you overcome the challenges stated above?

I would study until I knew a good amount of the material by myself first. Next, I would discuss those topics with others to reinforce what I knew vs what I had trouble grasping. I also learned to be available for myself as well. I did not completely swear off from having a life. I made sure that I rewarded myself with having fun or doing things that relaxed me.

5. What advice would you give a nursing student living on campus?

My best advice is to take advantage of all the resources on campus. Being able to study until times as late as 1-2 am in the library really helped me, especially when events are going on or people where partying. Try to master the art of time management. And lastly be available to have fun as well. Even the best of us can get burnt out, if we do not have time to recharge.

- Nassiwa Kayondo, BSN, RN

Interview with Thatiana Jeune BSN RN about living on campus experience

16. Did living on campus ease nursing school? If yes, explain how.

Living on campus did make going through the everyday difficulties of nursing easier. Having the ability to walk minutes to the library or the computer lab made working on homework, projects, and papers easier. To survive nursing school, you need to be able to organize your time efficiently and living on campus aided in that. Not having to factor commute time into my everyday tasks was great.

2. In your opinion, is living on campus more favorable for a nursing student?

I believe everyone has their preferences and what works for one may not work for all. Personally, for me living on campus did have its benefits but also its challenges and temptations. When living on campus it becomes difficult to escape the social aspects that comes along with it. If someone is focused and disciplined, then living on campus most definitely can be very favorable for a nursing student.

3. What challenges did you face as nursing student living on campus?

Some challenges I faced while living on campus is the temptations to join in on the social events going on. Although I was a nursing student I still did go to my schools events but I did have many situations where I really wanted to not study, or not work on that 10 page paper in order to go to "the party of the year". Having friends who were not in the nursing program who wanted you to go out did not make it any easier.

4. How did you overcome the challenges stated above?

Some of the ways I overcame the challenges above was by saying no and knowing that in the end my goal was more important. Another way I overcame this challenge was by planning ahead and balancing. For example, if I knew I had a paper due and there was also an event that I wanted to participate in I would make sure that I would get a certain amount of the paper done prior to going out. I know to some that may sound irresponsible, but although we are in college for our degree another huge component of college is being social and getting to know yourself. Obtaining both is possible if you manage your time properly and are focused.

5. What advice would you give a nursing student living on campus?

What I would tell a nursing student living on campus is use the benefits of being so close to all your resources such as being five minutes from the library, being able to schedule one on ones with your professors or tutors on campus, and not having to factor in the commute time. *Also, even though being a nursing student is very demanding do not deprive yourself of the full college experience.*

-Thatiana Jeune

Figuring out your finances and cutting unnecessary expenses is half the battle solved. In nursing school, *expenses are high while the funds are low.* I recommend that you sit down and review your financial plan before entering the nursing program that way you are better prepared to approach any inconsistencies in the future. Managing your finances will save you a lot eventually.

CHAPTER 4

Researching Accreditation and Addressing Legal Matters

Searching For A School That Is Certified And Accredited

After you have assessed your individual financial situation, shop around for a school that is within your perceived affordable budget. The school should not only be affordable, but it should also be able to equip you with a plethora of knowledge and most importantly, be ACCREDITED. You want to invest in a good school because at the end of the day, you are going to pay back the loans. No one wants to service a loan after having received a mediocre education or a useless diploma. Do not let your need to save lead you to a substandard school. Some nursing schools are on the verge of cancellation/closure, but they will still take new students and then let them go three quarters through school and they end up closing before students receive their diplomas. Do your research. Research the passing rates for the schools then compare. Is the school accredited?

It is important that you research the passing rates for schools before you enroll. These rates are very telling and will impact your own success while enrolled at that school. I have heard of students going through rigorous programs only to fail the NCLEX exam multiple times because of lack of preparation. A school with a good pass rate is more likely to prepare you to pass the NCLEX on the first attempt. While you shop around for a school, keep that in mind. The pass rates are a good indicator of success.

Accreditation

One of the most important points to consider when locating a school is whether it is accredited. There are two types of accreditations for nursing schools. Accreditation Commission of Education in Nursing (ACEN) and Commission on Collegiate Nursing Education (CCNE). These accreditations are in place to ensure that schools meet all standards in training professional nurses. Some schools are open and run a curriculum but are not yet accredited because accreditation is voluntary. Enrolling in a nursing school that is accredited has its benefits. Nursing students can transfer credits within the state and nationally, take the licensure exam, and further your education.

Do your research, look up pass rates and read up on any substantial information before considering enrollment. There are consequences to enrolling in schools that are not accredited. You might not be able to take the board exam. Sometimes it also affects your ability to further your education because the standard of education you received at the said school is below state and national requirements. Get familiar with the types of accreditation, how you can be affected as an individual, and decide whether you want to go through the trouble. I am anal about getting information from the right sources. Google is great. However, one should get into the habit of physically visiting the schools, arranging to speak to students that are enrolled or were enrolled in the school. Asking someone you know is not good enough. Visit the nursing board sites, attain numbers and emails, and reach out to the right resource.

Important questions to ask while reviewing accreditation include learning how many years the school has been accredited. It is important to know because, if a school was granted accreditation in the year of 2017, only the students during the same year and those that follow are considered to have attended an accredited nursing program (ACEN, 2017).

Is the school you are considering under review? Schools are continually evaluated to ensure they meet the criteria as stipulated by the commission (ACEN, 2017). To search for an accredited nursing school, go to the ACEN website under "search for accreditation." You will need to enter information for the state, program, and institution. The search will yield the accredited schools, the date of first accreditation, next visit, stipulations, and the program administrators. You can also visit the CCNE website for the same search.

According to the ACEN website, as of the year 2017, accreditation is required from admission to graduate level. If continuing your education is in your future, these are the questions you should be asking yourself and the advisors before you commit. Learn more about the process for 56ransferring credits from one school to another. Gather more information on accountability of schools, which ensures that the faculty are qualified and credentialed to achieve the desired education outcomes. ACEN also provides students with information on recruitment and a school's ability to receive funding from the state and federal agencies (Accreditation Commission for Nursing Education, ACEN,2017). *ACEN and CCNE is to colleges what JCAHO is to health facilities.* Both organizations hold institutions to a certain level of accountability.

ACTION TOOL

- After locating a school, search the school in the Accreditation Commission for Education in Nursing (ACEN) database.
- What entry level of nursing are you considering?
- Know the difference between ACNE and CCNE. According to a blog post by RN Careers, CCNE accredits bachelor's and master programs whilst ACNE accredits practical to doctorate entry levels of nursing and works hand in hand with the government to provide financial support (Differences between CCNE and ACNE, RN Careers, 2019). It then comes down

to what level of education, you are seeking and your financial need.

- Determine the entry level you are interested in. Self-assessment is key.

Entry Level

A friend of mine who had just completed her licensed practical nursing (LPN) program confessed that she would not be able to pursue a BSN, RN immediately because after assessing herself and capabilities, she believed that she needed more time practicing as an LPN before advancing her career. It is important to know what your limitations are, and how you plan to break through them. Years later, she is now enrolled in an RN bridge program. Some people prefer to complete tasks one at a time and not all at once. If nursing is for you, you will certainly find a way.

The beauty of nursing is that there are several entry levels. These several entry levels include: Certified Nursing Assistant, Licensed Practical/Vocational Nurses, Associates Degree in Nursing, baccalaureate prepared nurses and accelerated nursing programs, which are pursued by individuals with bachelor's degrees in related fields. The choice of entry is dependent on who you are, the amount of time each program takes to complete, commitments outside of school, financial, and social support, and much more. That is why you should evaluate all these aspects before deciding. Nursing programs are rigorous and require the individual to be motivated to succeed. Being highly motivated aligns with preparedness.

I know many nurses that started out as licensed practical nurses and now have doctorates in nursing. The pros of nursing are that you can build upon your education. I personally started out as a certified nursing assistant and pursued an Associate Degree in Nursing (I) only to end up in a baccalaureate degree program because I wanted to do it all at once. I am now considering a doctorate versus critical care NP. It is important that I have enough experience before pursuing a higher level of nursing.

Filter out the outside noise and assess yourself as an individual. What role do you want to play as a nurse? This is a clarifying factor and will guide you in making the right decision. One of my longtime friends struggled with the decision to either pursue licensed practical/vocational nursing (LPN/LVN) or BSN. She is now currently enrolled in BSN program. Her decision was simplified once she understood the roles involved, where she can practice and the opportunities therein.

It is helpful to find and speak to individuals already practicing in the fields you hope to pursue and decide if it is the right fit. Find a mentor. Follow their routine, observe their roles as well as their satisfaction in said roles. The time it takes to complete all these programs varies and so does the commitment. On average, an LPN program takes about one year to complete; the associates or I program takes two years; the BSN program takes four years; and the accelerated degree in nursing could take up to eighteen months, respectively. You need to have a health-related degree to pursue an accelerated degree in nursing.

Timelines to complete various entry levels of nursing

Entry Level	Requirements	Time	Licensure
Licensed Practical Nurse	Completion of Practical Nursing Diploma	Up to 12 months	Passing NCLEX-PN LPN also known as LVN
Associates Degree in Nursing	Completion of Associates Degree in Nursing Diploma	18 months-2years	Passing NCLEX-RN RN
Bachelor's in Nursing	Completion of Bachelor's in Nursing Diploma	4 years	Passing NCLEX-RN RN/
Accelerated Degree Bachelor's Degree Nursing (A nurse with a prior bachelor's degree in another health-related field.	Completion of pre-nursing requirements/classes. Completion of 16 months BSN program	16 months (As stated by Northeastern University in Boston Massachusetts)	Passing the NCLEX-RN RN/

Timelines may change over time. Consult with colleges of interest for credibility. The timelines stated are only applicable when one takes no breaks during school.

CLEP

For students that are coming from overseas or have completed courses at different colleges, you can attain credit toward some of the nursing pre-requirements through CLEP. CLEP stands for College

Level Examination Program. It tests students in various courses to enable them to gain credit in the courses they have already completed. Faculties at schools will then determine if the knowledge level assessed meets the requirements as taught at the school of choice. This is a route one can take to avoid retaking classes. Some classes, however, should be taken within the required amount of time. Classes such as chemistry and statistics should be taken within five years to apply for credit.

Again, before considering this route, make sure that the school accepts this credit. For more information on CLEP, the test structure, location, and courses, visit the CLEP site via clep.collegeboard.org (check the references section for further directions on accessing the site)

Have you practiced as a nurse in another country?

Nurses that have practiced in other countries also have an opportunity to continue their practice if they happen to move to the United States. Requesting information from the correct source is important. The NCLEX website offers a wealth of information regarding this query. Visiting your state's licensure board website is the first step towards getting clarity. *Always ask, never assume.*

Students from other countries that have completed nursing and/or have practiced outside the states can take the NCLEX examination along with a few classes to become licensed. The best source of information is the NCLEX website. Search for information related to licensure requirements for nurses that have practiced outside of the United States.

You have located a school. One that suits both your financial and educational needs, now what?

After you have located a school that meets all the criteria, the next thing you need to do is take a campus tour, meet with an advisor, and discuss all the expectations. Being clear and intentional right from the beginning will enable you to get exactly what you are looking to achieve. There are a couple of questions you must ask your advisor and tour guide, these include: where the library is; what time it closes; and what resources in the library are available to you (Because that will be your favorite place, trust me). Look for other available resources such as tutors, extra study space, and what time these places open and close. Knowing your resources and where to find them is crucial for any nursing student. We have extraordinarily little time to learn a lot of information and wasting that time locating things you could have done ahead of time is not ideal. Not only will preparation serve you well as a student, but it will also augment your nursing practice, as well as your life.

TOURING SCHOOLS

You are visiting the potential campus. Here are a few things to keep in mind while touring the school.

- Do a scavenger campus tour.
- Note your advisor's email, phone number, and find their office location.
- Locate the library (make sure to note hours of operation and reserve section for books), book store, cafeteria, private study spaces, tutors, nursing simulation labs, and gym.
- Locate the nursing organization on campus and enroll.
- Obtain a copy of the graduation requirements for your year of graduation. This is particularly important for students that have transferred into a new a school.

Addressing Legal Matters Before Choosing A School

As you will learn soon, this is a profession that is governed by a code of ethics. Your past in terms of legal matters is a huge component of it. I am mentioning this because you will not be able to practice as a nurse if these legal matters are not resolved. Things such as felonies, driving under the influence, and a criminal past are important to take care of before considering a profession such as nursing. If we must practice under the code of ethics, we must abide by the expectations therein.

Do you have a criminal background? Have you committed federal crimes, or do you have a DUI in your past? If the answer to any these is a yes, see that you settle these disputes prior to pursuing this career.

A lot of schools will request a background check but sometimes the background checks are not extensive enough. I know of people that have gone on to attend four years of school only to find out that they cannot take the board exam. Seek legal advice and inquire from the schools and the state board of nursing. Check if you are clear to go before spending lots of money and time only to find out that you are not legible to practice as a nurse.

Taking legal matters and accreditation into account before choosing a school is crucial. As mentioned in the chapter, this information might not be readily available to you. However, there are credible nursing sites you can utilize to find the most up-to-date information about the schools you choose to attend before wasting your time and resources. I would strongly advise against enrolling in a school that is on probation. Visit ideal schools ahead of time before making a choice. This is your education. You are entitled to the best.

CHAPTER 5

Learner and Personality Types and Concept Maps

―――――― o ――――――

What kind of learner are you?

A farmer will make sure that the tools he needs are with him
before heading out to the farm.

For those that know a little about farming, there are various garden
tools. Each tool was designed to only do the job it is meant to do.
For example, a garden fork cannot be used to dig. That is something
a garden hoe does, or a spade will not be used to plough and so on.
This concept can be applied to nursing students. How do you expect
to learn when you do not even know how best you learn? Before entry
into the program, one should have a clear understanding of their
learning needs. Learning needs will sometimes change during the
program. If this happens, you re-evaluate and take a different approach
and use trial and error to eliminate what works and what does not.

For a nursing student or any student for that matter, your way of
learning is what is going to keep you afloat in this rigorous program.
The amount of learning condensed in four years is a lot. To avoid

lagging select the learning tools that are specific to the way you learn. Some students are fortunate enough to be able to incorporate all learning methods. These are your brilliant individuals. The ones you love to hate. Like how do they just know it all? I can reassure you that once you know your learning tool and/or needs, you are bound to be successful. Ever wondered how smart students understand something almost immediately? Knowing how you learn increases your efficacy. Once you master your learning tool and utilize it, you will excel.

If you dive into nursing school without knowing what kind of learner you are, two things will happen. One, you waste a lot of time and must I remind you that nursing school waits for no man. Two, you discover later in the program what your strengths are, but then it is too late to turn back the hands of time. In this case, a stitch in time saves nine.

Considering the complexity of the information received during nursing school, the way you learn changes. I recommend not sticking to old learning habits especially if they have been unsuccessful. How do we know that what you are doing is not working? By giving it a first try, right?

After your first nursing exam, you will realize that you did not perform as well as you always have. I know of students that crammed everything prior to nursing school, and it worked. They were 'A' students then. Fast forward to their first nursing school exam, and they bombed it using the same techniques they thought would work. *You cannot cram 1000 pages of content. You must understand and apply it.* There you have it. If the way you study for an exam is not producing satisfactory results, change things up before it is too late.

Types of Learners

The VARK model identifies four types of learners: visual, aural/auditory, read and write and kinesthetic.

Table defining each learning type with examples

Visual	Aural/Auditory	Red and write	Kinesthetic
These learners learn by viewing	These learners learn by hearing or speaking	These learners learn by word usage	These learners learn by doing. Tactile learners fall under this category
Example: Utilize graphs, maps, symbols, flow charts (will excel with concept maps use)	Example: Utilize lectures, discussion groups, talk things aloud, record oneself	Example: Utilize PowerPoints, will excel at essay and written assignments	Example: Utilize clinical settings, simulations, case studies, videos, or movies

It is important to know how you process and learn unfamiliar information. I have learned that success in nursing school is based on one's ability to understand and apply content. Once you understand content, no matter how the question is thrown at you, you will prompt your brain for a solution. This will enable you to succeed later in the program when the content becomes more complex.

Do not waste time doing something that is not yielding results. If you have utilized a learning method and have found that you are not successful after several attempts, try a different learning method. Learning is meant to be fun. When you enjoy the way you learn, you begin to love learning. A tactile or kinesthetic learner for example, will thrive during clinical rotations where they are hands on with assignments because they learn best by touching and doing things.

Visiting simulation labs and practicing skills that are not experienced during rotation is also beneficial for this type of learner.

After receiving your acceptance into the program, you usually have a summer or winter break before the rigorous process begins. I recommend spending the summer prior to the start of the semester evaluating your learning methods. Believe me, this is going to work for you. You will discover that some of the ways that worked for you before are not as effective anymore. You cannot cram your way through nursing school. Every semester lays a foundation for the next semester, and if you are not able to apply the material from a previous semester, you will have trouble connecting the dots later.

Nursing school is like a big puzzle. The curriculum is organized in a way that enhances knowledge at every level. On completion of a class, you connect the dots with the class you took prior, and at the end of it all, you are to process information in bits to arrive at a solution.

Content is introduced in blocks. Block by block, you build a foundation. Anatomy and Physiology will teach you how the different body systems function, microbiology will focus on infectious agents, a pathophysiology class will then teach you the disease process and how the systems are affected by disease. You cannot comprehend pathophysiology if you did not take anatomy and physiology because first, you need to understand the normal function of a system. Just like, you cannot understand maternity if you have no idea what the anatomy of a woman looks like. Every class is a piece of the puzzle and as you progress, you put the pieces together. Your prerequisites are crafted to lay a foundation for what is to follow.

You will be required to take statistics, comprehension English classes, ethics, sociology, etc. All these classes are designed to turn you into a well-rounded nurse. If you are to go into research nursing, your statistics class will come handy. Your English classes will help you summarize, edit, and equip you with the narrative skills you will need for effective documentation. It is therefore important to know what learning tools you use because, as you can see, you are required to understand so many views in the same setting.

I am a combination of visual and read-write, but after I discovered that I had mastered the concepts, I realized I could apply them in the clinical setting (kinesthetic). This led me to believe that one can utilize all learning methods once they have mastered the content. To placate my learning, I watch a lot of videos. Thank God for Simple Nursing! If you are a visual learner, look up Michael Linares. He has several YouTube videos and a website with simplified content. He is great. Michael Linares is very articulate and has all these fun ways of presenting information that makes recalling easier. He also has multiple mnemonics and even songs.

If you are a visual learner, I recommend that you check him out. You can also follow his Instagram page; he posts picmonics to enhance learning, so you can continue to learn on the go. Speaking of picmonics, visual learners, there are multiple applications available to you. All you must do is search the web, your mobile apps and even consult with IT services at your schools to find out what is available to you. Remember to utilize and exhaust ALL your resources.

When I study, I write down or highlight the important points. Don't we all? *A highlighter is a nursing student's best friend.* This habit also classifies me as a read-write learner. There are multiple ways to exhaust this type of learning as well. One can make flash cards for complex scientific terms, drugs, and mnemonics. When I found that I did not have a piece of paper and pen, I would write in the notes section of my iPhone then rewrite the information on paper later. Endeavor to exhaust all the tools in your vicinity. Think freely, get creative with learning.

Thinking freely and being creative in finding a solution is the art of nursing. You always want to learn and do things different because the truth is; there is more than one way to do things. There are a lot of things you can use. Once you know what your learning method is, read more about it and find ways to be creative with it. You will find that learning is so much fun after that. I love learning. One of the reasons I do, is that I love the way I learn. So, exhaust all the learning tools that fit your learning style. There is a lot of content out there. Use it.

All your PowerPoint presentations and chapter introductions have learning objectives. This is the material your instructor expects you to know when you finish reading that chapter. You have fully integrated that information if you can answer the learning objectives in depth without opening a chapter or your notes.

After I study, I test myself using question banks such as Saunders NCLEX review and read the rationales. When I continuously fail a certain disease process, procedure, or technique, I review that material again and test myself to affirm that I have learned the material. The beauty in testing oneself is that you learn diverse ways of how the information will be assessed on an exam. The questions also redirect you to what is important to know. Reading rationales on questions will also teach you how to think like the examiner.

Book chapters are filled with useful information, but not all that information is important to know. You will find that doing multiple questions will clue you into what is important to know. Questions are frequently asked to reiterate what is important to know. If you understood a subject, you can apply in so many ways. To assess your knowledge level, continue to test yourself.

Closer to the exam, I review my notes, review PowerPoint presentations, and test myself some more. You would rather score low prior to taking your test than have a low-test score on a real test. Test yourself before taking the test/exam.

For an auditory learner, the classroom is your initial learning environment. Auditory learners learn by listening. To maximize your retention of material, review topics ahead of class. This will help you process information as it is relayed to you. Another tool you can utilize is recording the lecture and replaying it a later time. If you plan to record a lecture, make sure you notify your instructor and request permission. The market is saturated with resources to enhance your learning. Your job is to know what works best for you. Sitting at the front of the class to avoid destruction is also a great idea for this type of learner.

Education is one of our roles as nurses. When you are creating patient care plans, you will have to assess the patient's learning needs and barriers to learning. You can utilize this knowledge (learning about your owning learning needs and barriers) in assessing how patients learn and retain information. Patients can teach back when they have retained information. As a student nurse, teach back is also as effective for an aural/auditory learner. Teach someone what you have learned.

The idea is that if you can teach back the information, you prove that you have learned it. You have become more knowledgeable and you have understood the material. To assess your knowledge about anything, teach someone. It is not a waste of time. One, you retain the information and two, you verbalize it and become confident with the material.

Choosing the Perfect Time to Study

You will find that during certain times of the day, your concentration is at its highest point. So, your task is to find out when you learn best. I have come across students that grasp content in the night, evenings and after midnight. My peak time is the wee hours of the morning. I plan my day to accommodate my wakefulness at 3 am in the morning. You must know the times that work best for you, and then you can plan your daily activities to accommodate your study time. Because I studied in the wee hours of the morning, I slept at 8 pm and the most sleep I would get was anywhere between 6-7 hours.

If you plan to work during school like I did, fit your study time into the schedule. Since I learned best in the wee hours, I worked overnight shifts. I would go to school during the day, sleep after classes and go to work at 8 pm or 7 pm for 12 hours shifts. I had a gap before classes, so I would recuperate, attend class, and repeat the cycle. Planning your time and sticking to your schedule is vital. Never procrastinate even though we do, and I did. Procrastination is a vice. This is what sparks your blood pressure and increases your anxiety. In turn, you are less productive and less focused. Discipline is crucial in maintaining the work-school balance.

I worked full-time and I was still able to meet my academic expectations. How did I do it? By being disciplined and adhering to schedules. We all are not the same. I would advise that you listen to your body and do only what you can handle. And if you have help, take it. If your parents are supporting you through school, you do not have to work to meet your needs. Take all the help you can get.

Group Study

If you are a student that is into discussion groups, limit the number of participants to two or three. The more the number, the more time wasted contesting information. With a smaller group, you are more focused and agree to disagree much faster. And when you do disagree, you can consult the textbook and other sources.

Small groups are more effective. Being able to work in a group also will equip you with the interpersonal skills you will need in your professional role. Nursing is an interdisciplinary profession and learning to work well with others is a requirement for success. I think the purpose of group work in nursing school is to introduce team work and collaboration because nursing is an interdisciplinary profession.

Adhere to Successful Habits

Once you find something that works for you, stick to it. If it is not broken, why fix it? I found that reviewing material before major exams spiked my test scores. I always did one final review the morning of. For example, I scored 97% on a maternity test, which was a direct result of using this technique for the first time. This then became a habit. Before the exam, my friend and I went over what we thought was important. This resulted in both of us earning higher test scores.

Learning by Teaching and Concept Mapping

To learn, make use of your clinical rotations, continuously practice, teach, and question deviations. Another way of learning and retaining nursing interventions is by teaching patients in your rotations and have them teach back. You are learning and becoming proficient in teaching at the same time.

Concept mapping helps you retain complex information in nursing school. I did mention that nursing school is one huge puzzle that pieces lots of information together. Learning how to concept map can be an effective tool any learning type can utilize. It is also ideal for visual learners. They can place links to videos in the concept maps and revisit the links while studying. There are links from several YouTube sites that explain procedures, interventions, and so much more. Make concept maps work for you by incorporating yourself and the way you learn. Your concept maps are what you make them.

Concept map for nursing school success

Your brain is a map of sorts. Concept maps cluster information in terms of their level of importance, and your brain is tasked to place this information where it belongs for retrieval later.

Concept maps will get you through nursing school. This I can guarantee. Not only do they get you through, but they also enable you

to think as a nurse should. As students, we have a lot of information thrown at us in a short time. The only way to retain this information and make skillful use of it is by clustering it according to importance.

The typical concept map formulated by my nursing school consists of; risk factors, pathophysiology, signs and symptoms, labs and diagnostic tests, surgical and treatment modalities, medications, nursing diagnosis and interventions. One important thing to remember is to list the interventions in the order of importance. Think ABCs first and everything that follows. Listing the interventions in this manner will enable you make the right selections on your exams because your best answer is always going to be the highest priority.

The only way you will learn to think critically is by learning how to compartmentalize information in the order of importance. At the beginning of this book, I asked you why you chose nursing school. Your reasons are valid and should motivate you to work toward the end goal. The goal of nursing school, however, is for every one of us to be able think critically and prioritize when presented with a complex patient. Critical thinking is developed by having an adequate knowledge base, coupled with the right application.

The beauty of concept maps is that they can look the way you want them to. Incorporate your learning style in the concept maps to enable you to recall information quicker.

Refer to your learning style when creating a concept map. If you are a visual learner, plug in that cartoon character that signifies a concept. For example, Johnnie Bravo looks like he has lipodystrophy or Cushing's syndrome; Patrick from Sponge Bob has fluid overload signs and symptoms (classic ascites). Whatever helps you recall, use it.

Think creatively and make learning fun. I spent a lot of time creating concept maps for medical/surgical conditions and maternity/pediatric conditions, and I will tell you that it paid off. I used these same concept maps to review for NCLEX, and I still have them neatly tucked away someplace.

The other thing is that your concept map is structured for you. One cannot use your concept map and achieve the same results because they are unique. I would strongly advise that you review your learning mechanism and incorporate it in the concept maps. Create one template for disease processes and one for procedures and print these templates and insert information. Writing things down helps to recall them later.

Concept maps also cluster information according to importance. A critical thinker eliminates information based on importance. So, what are you waiting for? Concept map your way through nursing school. I always was asked how I know so much about a certain topic. I tell you; it is those damn concept maps. Start now, and you will not regret having started.

How to Create a Concept Map

Concept map for a disease process

1. Define the disease using key terms. You will have questions that include key terms that are specific to an illness without telling you what condition it is. A patient with right-sided heart failure will have ascites and dependent edema from third spacing, and impaired liver function because the liver is engorged. While a patient with left sided heart failure will show classic pulmonary congestion signs and symptoms to differentiate the two. Knowing these key differences in conditions will focus your interventions as a nurse. If you love to highlight, mark the differences in conditions.

2. Who is at risk? Eliminate the usual (smoking, obesity, etc.) Focus on what makes the risk factors unique to this disease process.

3. What are the signs and symptoms? Be specific. Focus on the signs and symptoms that only depict this disease process.

4. What are the specific lab results and tests? What will confirm this disease process? It is important to also note the differential diagnoses. (What else can mirror this disease process?) The look a likes.

5. What are the first line medications?

6. Write down nursing interventions in order of priority (ABCs, assessment before intervention). If your interventions include; fluid resuscitation, applying oxygen, assessing body systems, start with the intervention that is critical to prolonging life. It is always airway (oxygenation, elevating head of the bed, protecting the airway, intubation, etc.)

7. What could go wrong? How will you intervene? Always think ABCs.

Create a concept map for all the medical or surgical conditions using this template.

Next create a concept map for procedures, listing the procedure and purpose, complications from the procedure, nursing interventions in the order of priority, and after care for the procedure. Again, highlight what makes this procedure unique.

Because you need a video of how to concept map, I will create a YouTube video catered specifically to this.

Learning by Personality/behavior Types

If you find it harder to pay attention in the back of the class, sit at the front. I love sitting in the front seat. I do not know about the schools you go to, but we always chose our semester seats at the start of the semester.

On the first day of school, arrive early and sit wherever you please and that will forever be your seat. There will be students that forget the seats they self-assigned to themselves and cause havoc switching seats all semester. Students will recognize that it is your self-assigned seat and they will just leave you to it.

Personality and character types are also going to clue you into what mechanisms to manipulate to be successful in nursing school. If you have a type B personality, it would be smart to pair up with a type A personality. A type A is an individual that is highly organized and goal oriented. These individuals will push you to become better. Learning their ways will turn you into a successful student yourself. Pair yourself with what you seek to become. Choose your nursing school colleagues with caution. It is wiser to form mutualism relations where you benefit from one another. You never want to be caught in a parasitic relationship. This is a relation where only one benefits from the relationship. Consider the benefits of the company you keep.

Not only are we to assess patient and conditions, but we should also become experts of self-assessment. We as individuals should know who we are, what we are and what works best for us. That way, we can maximize all the resources in our vicinity. This is what I mean when I say the nursing school has taught me so much about life, everything that I learned is applicable in the real world.

The main goals of nursing school are to become critical thinkers and to learn how to prioritize. Before we become proficient in the former, we need to learn the basics and knowledge and then apply correctly. Knowing ones learning types, personalities and behaviors that increase learning will not only save time but enable us to succeed in this intense program. Take the test exercise on the VARK learning types to find out how you learn and then begin to utilize resources that support your learning type.

Assessment is a nurses' strongest suit. Assessing oneself will also strengthen your understanding and help you learn more about how important it is to gather information before partaking in anything. Through assessment of self, finances, schools, readiness for the program and learning needs, we have gathered enough information to create a plan that will enable us to succeed in the program. After assessment, we plan. In the next chapter, I will show you how to use all the information we gathered to create a working plan. But before we plan, we diagnose.

CHAPTER 6

Eliminating Distractions and Forming Strategic Nurse-Friendships

———————○———————

Halt the Party, Up the GPA

But you must always remember, it is not always about the
GPA, it is about how much you retain at the end of the day.

I n this chapter, I introduce student nursing diagnosis. Diagnosis is a
part of the nursing process. The nursing process includes;
Assessment, Nursing Diagnosis, Planning, Implementing and
Evaluation. We also are learning to apply the nursing process by using
simple examples. You will use the nursing process in care plans to drive
care. Introducing this concept now helps you to become familiar with
forming diagnosis'.

During diagnosis, we self-assess and state a problem or risk we are
more likely to encounter in nursing school and then plan to counteract
the problem. The concept of "student nurse" diagnoses is to list
common problems faced by nursing students worldwide. In stating the

problems, we then utilize other parts of the nursing process to work through the problem and hopefully solve it.

Student Nurse Diagnosis #1: Lack of a social life related to intensity of the program as evidenced by high GPA requirements, high pass rates, frequent exams/tests heavy course work load, etc.

"I have no life," says every nursing student. No. You have a life and nursing school is only but a tiny portion of your life. You will live after it. What is a year or two or even four years of your life? Not even a half of a whole. You will live. Buckle your seat belt because you are in for a ride.

Oh, the irony! Authoring a book to benefit nursing students as if they do not have enough on their plate already. Well, that may be right, but this is an action-oriented book. I intend to teach you something you never knew before to ease your nursing journey.

In this chapter, I will show you how to plan and implement. We need to plan out everything including the friends we chose, and how we are to balance work and school, while we are maintaining perfect grades and learning.

Halt the party. Or your GPA will suffer the consequences. There is plenty of time to party and "live" after nursing school. If we were to compare nursing school to growth and development stages, we are toddlers at the end of nursing school. That is, if you are enrolled in a four-year school. After nursing school, you will have plenty of time to party. You have your whole life to decide when to party, when to engage with your friends and catch up on everything you missed.

There is plenty of time to live your life after school, so buckle up and enjoy the rough ride. Nursing school is temporary.

Right now, you are excited about finishing nursing school. You are a nursing major and that means you really must put in time and effort to succeed. *A nursing degree is EARNED not given.* You must work hard. As a nursing major, you are serious from the get-go. You slack, you fail. You may have been told that your college life would be nothing but fun. They lied. Not for a nursing major. Maintaining a certain GPA keeps you enrolled in the program.

There is this quote I saved on my computer as my screensaver to pick me up when I was simply over it. The quote states:

"You are not studying to pass exams; you are studying for the day your knowledge level will be the only thing that will save your patient in a life and death situation."

— Unknown

I always needed some sort of affirmation getting through school as a nursing major. I would soak in affirmations and manifestations. So, find a quote that refocuses you and plaster that shit everywhere. On your phone or computer screensaver, in your car, dorm room...EVERYWHERE.

The classes you are taking at the beginning must sound like a cakewalk, don't they? However, do not underestimate the journey. These classes are your foundation, just as a blueprint is to a building. Passing the NCLEX in 75-questions begins in your first nursing class. Work hard now, do less later. Each one of those classes is a guide and a foundation for the next class to be built upon. The sooner you realize this, the better it is for you.

Nursing school is also equivalent to depositing money in the bank. With every deposit, there is an increment in the available funds saved up. All the classes you are taking are deposits of knowledge, which represent the information you will have to dig up later to understand topics in the future. If you made no knowledge deposits in the beginning, you will have to work three times as hard to stay afloat.

Plan to raise your GPA early in the program so that there are little to no surprises. The classes in the beginning are usually easier to pass, which means plan to have straight A's. A lot of us will struggle with a class and you never know which class will drop your GPA. So, make sure you excel at the easy classes. For many, anatomy and physiology or pharmacology is a challenge. That said, I do not mean that you should prepare to fail. I mean be prepared anyway.

Preparation, as you will learn, is key. Learn to anticipate things before they happen, prepare to counteract the problem should it occur. When you get into practice, anticipating a complication after surgery will save your patient because you will catch it before it kills or debilitates the patient. This is good practice.

Your first year as a nursing major is also equivalent to being benched for a game. You are not there yet. You have not even made "THE TEAM" and you must prove yourself before being accepted into the program. A lot of students do less during this time and have regrets later. Like I said, I will give you the tips. You decide if you want to follow through. A smart student will take these tips and make the most out of them and be more strategic.

Do not let nursing school play you, you play nursing school. Stay ahead and there will be no catching up later.

I am always in the library. Call me the library rat. My friends outside of nursing school always joked about my whereabouts and often said to others, "You always know where she is. Check the library first." On my many nights in the library, I met a first-year student. She was in the library as much as I was. I could tell she was going to be remarkably successful in the program. She was going as hard in the first year. We struck up a conversation, and when she realized that I was a senior in nursing school, she sought my advice on how to make it through nursing school. Uh huh! She and a lot of others are the reasons why I am authoring this book. This first-year student, however, is off to a good start. I told her a lot of what I will reveal in the book. Keep reading.

If partying is a distraction. It is time to stop the partying and focus. You cannot be out every weekend and expect to have a 4.0 at the end of the semester, unless of course you are a genius, but things do not always work like that. Being a committed student pays off at the end of the semester. Then you get to spend your break whichever way you want to and party till you drop or whatever floats your boat.

I always told myself that there is a life after nursing school. This sentiment has held my head up on days when I felt like it was simply too much for me to take. Construct a sentiment that will hold you together when you fall apart. You can adapt mine if it works for you. It worked for me.

All work and no play makes for a miserable student. Do not forget to have fun, but that is after taking care of the important things. First ask yourself, are all my assignments done? Have I prepared for the next class and did I understand all prior material? If the answer to all those questions is yes, then let loose. What you just did was prioritize. You eliminated the priorities to allow yourself some free time.

This is the beginning of a journey you will never forget. Going through nursing school is a whirlwind of emotions. In truth, nursing is hard! No surprises here. You are being trained to deal with human lives. That requires a lot of expertise, so before it is easy, it must be hard, and you will want to give up, but do not. I will walk you through the best way I know how. Old brooms know all the corners. You can trust that I have encountered a few things to pass on.

SPOILER ALERT! Partying hard and nursing school do not go together. If you do, you might just fail out faster than you picked it up. So, decide what is more important; a party that will end in a few hours or a career? The thing about parties is that they will always be there. Weigh your options. Know your priorities. Those who love you will understand why you are never available to engage. It takes challenging work to build a nurse.

Fast forward to the future. I wrote this chapter in nursing school. After having done everything I speak of in this chapter, I am being inducted into the nursing honor society and graduating with honors. Yes, I fell short of magna cum laude by .225 points, but that is simply fine. I know that challenging work pays off and it feels so damn good. Get to work. This will be you soon. Now I have all the time in the world to party.

The friends you keep in nursing school will make or break you. Deciding to eliminate friends that do not mirror your hard work and values is important. Sometimes the behaviors we adapt in nursing school are influenced by the company we keep. Forming friendships with individuals that have shared goals suppresses the need to impress those with unfamiliar goals. We explore why in the following section.

Forming Strategic Friendships/Nurseships

Part of excelling in nursing school requires one to choose the RIGHT nursing school friends. It sounds selfish but at the end of the day, it serves you. Forming strategic relationships/nurseships helps you eliminate distractions. In this section, explore the importance of your choices and how they affect you in the program.

Plan: Strategically choosing friends with shared goals and interests to keep you focused through nursing school.

Everyone needs a friend. In life, you will find that you always gravitate toward people that are most like you. Similar interests, tastes, backgrounds, cultures, and what not. In nursing school, you must put more thought into the friendships you make. These friends will make or break you.

Student nurses need strategic friendships. Forming strategic friendships can alleviate the requirements of the program. By pairing yourself with strong students, you cut your work in a half. How? Their strength will not only be your motivation, but it will also help you to model the same attributes they possess. I learned the importance of being organized from one of my closest friends. This helped me to relive the stress that comes with due dates and instructor requirements.

Choosing friends that have shared interests will also counteract peer pressure. Sometimes people do things because friends influence them. If the friends you chose are focused on excelling in nursing school, you will be focused too. If they are party animals, you will be a party animal. Strategize, choose wisely.

I mentioned earlier that your friendships should be mutual, meaning you should be benefiting from the friendship. Avoid parasitic relationships especially in nursing school. You cannot afford to waste time helping someone else when you should be helping yourself. That is, unless you are an extraordinarily strong student. And by strong, I mean scores above 95% on every exam. Help yourself first then assist another.

Time is not of the essence in nursing school. Therefore, forming friendships is an important task you must complete early on. If you are a weak student, pair yourself with a strong student. Please have something to offer in return. Do not become a parasite. Work on your strengths and bring something to the nurseship. Soon enough you will learn their ways, and before you know it, you will be stronger than you were before.

Successful students have habits. These are habits that you are looking to emulate. If you are a very disorganized person, pair yourself with an organized individual. This individual will keep you updated about what tests or assignments are due. Know your weaknesses and look to pair yourself with someone who is stronger in those areas.

I know of people that formed nurseships and went on to become lifelong friends. This goes back to assessment. Assess yourself as an individual and determine what your strengths and weaknesses are. Then draw or seek to attract the people that will strengthen your weaknesses while you hopefully do the same for them. Should you sense that the nursing relationship is more of a burden that does not benefit you, halt the relationship early on.

Nurseships should also include a professional network. They are referred to as nurse mentors. Find nurses practicing in the field that can guide your steps and reassure you that there is a light at the end of the tunnel. When you have a problem regarding the profession, you will be able to consult with your professional network about it. Only people that have gone through the program understand, and people in your network can also refer and connect you to job opportunities when you graduate. Instagram and YouTube is another source of nursing inspiration. There are lots of nurses that are giving advice on YouTube and Instagram. Find these pages and use them to uplift your spirit and motivate you.

Nurseships are incredibly unique friendships because they consist of people of nursing with shared interests and sometimes goals. Only we understand the struggle. Most times, people on the outside will not understand why you are always busy and why you never make it to a family event and/or gathering. You might lose friends, grow distant from family, and sometimes break off relationships because they become a distraction. A fellow nursing student or nurse gets it, if they have not been there, they know someone that has, and their support is more than valuable. Be sure to create a network of people like you.

Using Checklists to Help You Choose Strategic Friendships/Nurseships

We must learn how to be successful in finding our strategic friendships. This will help equip you for success. One way to do this is by filling out checklists. I love checklists! They narrow things down to what is essential to do/know. Now we will utilize checklists to choose nurseships.

By using checklists, you will learn to group information in brief context and only include the task followed by an action. Once you check something off, consider that done. Despite how much we try, we will never be able to recall everything we learned or plan to do. Checklists are an effective way of ensuring that most of the requirements are meant, tasks are completed, and we will start to explore how best to use them early on using simple information like; checklists for a desired nurseship. By the time you graduate from nursing school, you will be an expert in the use of checklists and will be able to complete nursing tasks in simple steps.

Have you ever gone to the grocery store with a list of items you were prepared to buy prior to leaving the house versus going to the store without one? The difference is when you make a list, you are more likely to get all the items you were looking to buy and save money because you are not buying unnecessary items. I honestly need a checklist for my trips Target because without one, I assume I need everything. When you commit to memory, you might forget to get an item you intended to get.

Checklist for desired nurseship

- Assess the relationship even before it begins. Does the friendship meet your needs?
- In Chapter 1, you completed a through self-assessment, learning needs and diagnosis. Choose friends that learn like you do.
- Determine what their goals and expectations are. Are they like yours?
- If you are to choose social friends, make sure they at least care to work hard enough to make it out of school. Is your social life important to you? There should be a balance between academia and social life.
- Strong people will strengthen you; weak people will weaken you. Do you consider yourself as a strong or weak student? (Be honest).
- Personality types. Type A or Type B? What makes for a good working relationship? What is my personality type compared to my nurse-friend(s)? Research personality types. Myers-Briggs Personality Types theory can assist you in finding out what a personality type is. There are also other multiple theories that delve deeper into personality types and how

effective they can be if used in choosing friends, professions and much more.

- You have picked nurse-friend(s). This is your go-to support system. How supportive are they?
- Follow inspirational nursing pages on social media

1. Use the Myers-Briggs Personality Type Test to find out what your personality is.

_____

_____

_____

_____

2. Based on your responses, read up on your personality type and determine compatibility in choosing friends, profession and more.

Eliminating distractions such as partying and friends that do not fulfill the purpose of nursing school, will cut your work in a half, and allow you to utilize your time wisely. Learning to self-diagnose and identify problems you are most likely to face allows you to prevent or solve those problems ahead of time. We will continue to explore other student nurse diagnoses in proceeding chapters to not only solve problems but to learn how to utilize the nursing process by applying them to yourself.

CHAPTER 7

Student Nurse Tension and Support Groups

Student Nurse Tension

In the previous chapter, we explored how partying and choice of friends can impact nursing school grades. In this chapter, we will talk about student nurse tension and the support groups you will need to help you approach these situations better. I utilize the nursing process yet again and state a student nurse diagnosis and produce a plan to counteract the problem. Again, using the nursing process casually to address common student nurse problems enhances your prowess in the use of the nursing process.

Student Nurse Diagnosis #2: At risk for student nurse bullying related to program requirements as evidenced by student nurse tension, competitiveness, and high attrition rates of certain ethnic backgrounds due to lack of support and lateral violence.

Bullying is one of the most ridiculous things that happen in nursing school that unfortunately makes its way into practice. Student nurses look at each other as competition, which is reasonable but cruel.

We all compete to pass classes and meet selection requirements, and in the process develop cruel habits. Some nursing students develop habits like; the withholding of vital information and distributing false information in hopes to derail others and sometimes set each other up for failure.

This is a subject that needs some attention. I want to help you counteract this problem should it occur. Part of being a successful student is being able to anticipate problems and plan to avoid the problem. I will highlight my thoughts that derive from a lived experience. My hopes are that you can identify the student nurse tension and that you choose to act differently.

Competition is the norm in nursing school, but it should never harm others. It is great but not that great of a tool since it creates so much tension, division, and creates habits that then resurface in health care practice.

We must realize that even though we are competing to survive and stay above required scores, nothing is more detrimental to teamwork than tension amongst your colleagues. Nursing school is supposed to teach us both the art and science of nursing. Communication and relating with others (art of nursing I believe) are not only essential to nurse-patient relationships but also to nurse-to-nurse relationships and then nurse-organization relationships. Continuing to partake in these behaviors creates a foundation for nurse bullying, lateral violence, etc.

We must learn earlier that we can all co-exist and one's knowledge level in no way diminishes yours. We are incredibly unique and whatever we bring to nursing as individuals is valuable. Celebrating and learning from others' strengths makes one better. Therefore, do not feel threatened by the next individual. Perfect your art or science and strengthen nursing. Focus on your own personal and professional growth.

I always thought that most of the vices in practice originate from nursing school. The behaviors we learn to accept early on become the norm in the future. There are nursing units in practice that are toxic work environments. Nurses on these units are continuously plotting against each other and bullying others out of practice. Saying no to nurse bullying right from the get-go as a student and always speak up for the ones that are being bullied into silence. How can we practice healing when we are ourselves are broken? Or are breaking others? We should apply the paradigm of nursing first to ourselves and then to others. Be the change you want to see in the nursing world. Decide today as a nursing student not to take part in any form of bullying and to always speak up for others.

Programs have been set up to create this kind of tension. The truth is that if one works hard enough, they will make it. The American Nurses Association has echoed that there is a constant need for nurses. That is affirmation that there's room for everyone. This crab in the barrel mentality has negatively impacted teamwork and collaboration and has even led to the premature exit of students from programs and the nursing profession.

We as future nurses are all working toward the same goal. We have shared goals. In nursing school, our collective goal is to become nurses. In practice, our goal is to positively impact patient lives. So, it is important to realize early on that we are stronger together and the more cohesive a group is, the more likely it is to succeed.

If you are already experiencing this alienation or tension, my advice is that you stay far away from these behaviors. Make friends with a few students, respect each other, and assist one another in any way you can. Also, make sure to notify the student body about students that partake in bullying behaviors.

I am sure that some of you are working in places where you have witnessed nurse-to-nurse bullying. The root of this is in nursing school. Students have been known to create divisions such as: the brilliant ones, the weak, the smarter, the pretty ones, the black students, the white students, etc. Do these dichotomies sound like team work and collaboration to you?

In my senior year, I came to realize that we all deserved to be there, and I was very respectful of other students. I looked around and realized that despite how divided we were in the beginning, we all deserved to be there. A working solution to student-nurse tension is support groups. In the next section we explore why support groups are essential to one's survival in nursing school.

Support Systems

Plan: Build a dedicated support system to reduce the chances of bullying, student-nurse tension, stress, etc.

Your success in nursing school depends on the foundation of your support systems. Who is holding you up when you are on the verge of quitting? Who is pouring positivity into you while when you are distraught with school?

While in nursing school, I thought the idea of implementing nursing support groups would be effective in relieving stress. As you will learn, nurses recommend support groups to patients with new and challenging diagnoses to help them cope with illnesses, body image concerns and so on. Nursing school is no different. The stress related to the program requires student nurses to learn new ways of coping and forming support groups is a working solution. It is with this same understanding that I attempted to exploit or create nursing support groups for nursing students.

If your school has none, make suggestions to implement one. It is true that only the people that have gone through or are going through nursing school will understand your frustrations. I came across a study that called support groups "care groups." Whatever you call them, these groups can be effective in subsidizing stress that arises from the program and create a cohesive group with shared goals.

Nursing Support Groups

Even though I was unsuccessful in fully implementing nursing support groups under my leadership of the nursing student body, I believe that every nursing student body should have a nursing support group dedicated to student nurses. These support groups can be further divided into groups of five students that perform activities together to alleviate stress. Activities can include yoga, paint nights, morning/evening runs, and discussions about issues incurred in the program.

The support groups can even include instructors and former students to guide and support existing students through the program. Reach out to your student governments and request that these support groups are in place to support you. I strongly believe in support groups and their ability to alleviate stress and cultivate new coping mechanisms. Make sure to join the student nursing organizations on campus, and in state and national organizations. There are a lot of resources available to student nurses. There are also nurse support groups on Face-book and Instagram. Join them as well.

Support Outside of Nursing School

Many of the students I know ended their relationships while in nursing school. The other half struggled in their relationships. Nursing school is stressful. If you are dating, your partner should be supportive. Many women and men meet their life partners in college. Balancing school and a relationship can be challenging, especially if you are enrolled in a rigorous program. Your partners are your backbone; they must be strong.

I come from a very traditional background and pursued nursing after the age of 22. A woman of that age in my background should be settled or at least have a strong suitor. Sometimes we are pressured to conform to societal norms and attempt to do it all. Times have changed. As I mentioned before, nursing school is only a portion of your life. You can meet someone at any point in your life. If a career is important to you, focus on it first.

The thing with nursing school is that it unravels you. I do not mean to scare you, but the partner you keep needs to understand the intensity of the program and what you are up against. Many nurses have built successful relationships that later lead to marriage but that takes a special kind of man or woman. Like I have continuously stressed, the only distraction you need is school. Anything that draws too much of your attention needs to go. If your partner is not going to be supportive, they might as well not be there.

I was dating in nursing school. The exhaustion of it all! I always could not go anywhere, and even when I managed to, I was tired. I recall sleeping at the movies, not cooking, doing laundry that was weeks old, eating poorly unless someone cooked… I can say now; it was all worth it. If I had to do it again, I would do it the same way.

This is an extremely rewarding career, and you are on the right path. Remember that when you are frustrated.

Friendships Outside of Nursing School

The friends you made prior to entry into the program will most likely become distant. The beauty is that you can reconnect during the summer and school breaks. But never let the pressure of "meeting up" with friends affect your education. True friendships will stand the test of time. Your friend's lifestyle will not exactly mirror yours but think about it, nursing school is a few years of your life, not your entire life, and this is a sacrifice you can endure.

If at all you feel let down, remind yourself why you started in the first place. I canceled commitments very often. Then my friends got to a point where they just did not ask me to do things anymore. I always told myself that this was a phase that would soon be over.

If you made great friendships, they will stick around no matter what and understand your predicament and support you through it all.

I have friendships I formed prior to nursing school that have stood the test of time. These friends were so encouraging. I remember posting a lot of library pictures, and they would encourage me. They were so supportive. Never underestimate the power of encouragement. Make friends that you know will always uplift you no matter what. And for the friends you make while in nursing school, those are friendships for life. Two of my favorite instructors were in nursing school together, worked together and just seemed to go where the other went.

Family Support

Family support is important. I come from a large family. I am one of twelve children. I know. See how many heartbeats I can listen to for practice? Your family is your God given support system. The support might be financial, emotional, or social. My youngest sibling was four years old at the time. Some days were very tough days and I just did not know how to carry on, and there was this little girl who asked if she could use my "stethoscope" to listen to my heart. Little things like these warmed my heart and always pushed me to want to do more. While I was learning, so was she. She always asked me about the sick people I took care of when I returned from clinical. Her interest in what I was doing really did inspire me.

I want you to know that your families will be/are proud of you. Even before you graduate from nursing school, they will come to you with health-related questions. They will tell anyone that cares to listen that their child is a nurse (even though you are technically not there yet). They will consult with you about cold therapies and whatever God knows they are ailing from. Draw from their enthusiasm and become what they have envisioned you to be. Their belief in you should empower you. I hope everyone of you has a family that supports your nursing journey. This will simplify the process.

And always reach out for support from them. Do not expect everyone to assume your needs. You are never alone. There are support systems in your school (financial, emotional, and social, at work, within the student body. There is a lot of support around you. Self-evaluate and reach out.

Support System Survey

1. What kind of support do you need (financial, emotional, social)?

2. What types of support systems do you have in place?

3. Do you work? Is your job supportive of your education? Find work that does not hinder your nursing education.

4. Are you in a relationship? Is it a supportive relationship? If not, reconsider.

5. Is your family involved and supportive?

6. Are your friends keeping you on the right track?

7. Is your faculty and study body supportive?

8. Does your school have nursing support groups?

Answer these questions honestly. Make it a point to research the resources available to you and use them to alleviate the stress that comes from nursing school.

Support groups are a working plan to eliminate the vices of student nurse tension and bullying. As mentioned in the chapter, these habits do make their way into practice. Recognizing these habits brings us one step closer to eliminating them. My hope is that this chapter has brought to light the importance of support groups (family, relations, and school) in nursing school.

CHAPTER 8

Work and School Balance

Working While In School

Another common student nurse problem is the balance between work and school. We again utilize the diagnosis part of the nursing process to formulate a student nurse diagnosis and form a working plan to eliminate presumed hardships as we have in the two previous chapters. Our approach to the work and school balance is to show how imbalance affects grades, increases stress, and derails time management. In this chapter, we make a plan that enables us to stay afloat.

Student Nurse Diagnosis #3: At risk for dropping out of school due to failure to balance work and school schedules as evidenced by poor performance both at work and school, and stress related to inability to meet deadlines.

Again, if you can afford it, do not work. If you must work, work in a health-related field. Working in the field is extremely helpful. The way I looked at working while in nursing school was, if I had to do it, it would have to be in an environment that enhanced learning.

Working at a hospital on a step-down telemetry floor was very hectic especially during school because I made a mistake and chose work requirements that were not conducive. I was required to work twelve hours a week and two weekends. My position was per diem but not flexible. You must choose a schedule that is flexible. This enables you to have some control of the schedule. Before accepting any position, make sure you understand the requirements. As you will find later, I did not see where I went wrong until I did, and I would like for you to not make the same mistake.

The plan therefore is to extensively review the work requirements therein to allow for flexibility. In the next section, we go over ways to ensure that there is a work and school balance that enhances learning and prevents stress related to inability to meet requirements.

Balancing Work And School

Plan: Balance work and school schedules. Choose work places and schedules that benefit you as a nursing student.

Choosing a Workplace

When you decide to look for work in a hospital, it is imperative that you review all the requirements therein. The most ideal is a monthly per diem position with flexibility. Never choose a fixed per diem weekly 12 or 24 because you will be required to work these shifts in a week.

With a monthly per diem position be it an 8-hour or 12-hour shift, you will be able to pick any day of the month to work and you can even pick more shifts when you are not burdened at school. You can also work more during school breaks because hospitals are always in need.

Create a good working relationship with your unit manager and scheduler and notify them that you are pursuing nursing school. I hope that they are very accommodating and if you find that they are not, look for work elsewhere. Your workplace needs to support your professional growth.

I chose the wrong work requirements (per diem 12 hour weekly with a requirement of two weekends a month) and had difficulty committing to this schedule as I was at school full time and during the weekends, I worked with a home health care agency. I could not forfeit school nor work. This arrangement was only sustainable in the first two years of nursing school. Once I started clinical rotations, it was exceedingly difficult to adhere to my previous schedule because I had to independently schedule 12 hours for clinical rotations. I found that I needed to cut back on work.

I thought to quit working at the hospital, but the benefits outweighed the risks. Then after assessing the pros and cons of working at the hospital, I chose to keep my hospital job because it enhanced learning.

Plan Ahead

You will have your syllabus at the start of the semester. At this time, sit down and with your planner, transfer all the important dates, highlighting test dates and due dates. After you have done this, pray that nothing changes because if it changes, that screws you up. If you work in a hospital, you will be required to put in all requests one month ahead of time. Set reminders before the requests are due so you never miss an opportunity to control your work/school schedule.

This practice will give you ample time to decide when you can and cannot work. This is something I should have put more emphasis on. Well, you know ahead of time now, so make it work.

I still hope that hospitals and other health facilities could devise a different scheduling system for nursing students. All these workplaces reiterate their commitment to continuing education, but not all of them have created environments that are conducive for student success. Perhaps create per diem status during school semesters and full time when students are not in school. A system such as this would allow for students to focus on school during the semester. Systems can be rigid and traditional in the ways they implement things, but change is pivotal and who knows what outcomes are to be achieved when we try a new way of doing things. Nursing students are a strong addition to health care systems, and they need to do a better job supporting them.

Why work during school?

"Iron sharpens iron." When you work in a hospital setting, the number of techniques you polish unknowingly are insurmountable. The students working in the field are a step ahead of their peers because they have a visual of disease presentation which makes it easy to recall signs and symptoms. I worked on a cardiac floor, and you could wake me up from sleep, and I would be able to talk about cardiac tests, nursing interventions, right-sided heart failure symptoms, etc.

The only downside to working in the field is that many times the practices in organizations are not up-to-date with NCLEX. Make sure to rely only on the material you are taught and not what you see in practice. Because NCLEX will test you by the book, not by practice. This does not mean that the practices in the field are wrong; it only means that you are tested differently. You will learn that you can never get too rigid about parameters such as vital signs, blood glucose, and electrolyte levels because they differ.

To harmonize work and school work in a field that contributes to nursing education. This includes all health care agencies. There are practices that benefit your education. I was lucky to get a job on a cardiac telemetry floor after my first clinical rotation.

This step-down surgery unit contributed to my nursing school. Working in this unit increased my knowledge level in cardiology as well as my passion for cardiology. I have worked with patients with various cardiac conditions. I was extremely comfortable with cardiology, signs and symptoms of cardiac conditions, procedures, and nursing interventions.

In my introductory nursing class, we were introduced to chest tubes, and like any other nursing students, I was not comfortable working with chest tubes. Working as a clinical care tech on a cardiac unit exposed me to a lot of chest tubes and with time, I was more knowledgeable and able to test with ease.

It is on this unit that I learned how to perform an EKG, read, as well as interpret one. My cardiac nursing classes were the easiest because I could relate to the content. I recommend that nursing students find work in the field. The amount of knowledge you attain is worth it. Matter of fact, if you find a system or subject difficult, find work in that same exact field. You will learn by association.

There was a time when I worked a total of 40 hours and was taking four courses. This is unheard of, and everyone I know wondered why I worked so hard despite being engaged in an intense program. I worked both at the hospital and in-home care. I was excelling in nursing school despite my work commitments. Preparation and strategy are vital when balancing work and school. Home care was not as demanding as working on the cardiac unit. While my patients slept, I stayed up studying and checked on them every 1-2 hours to meet their needs. Days are busy, and it is hard to catch a break. If you are looking to work a lot or are required to, plan on working nights and weekends as opposed to day shifts.

Invest in summarizing your class work into easily reviewable material. While working nights, I practiced taking tests and I made my drug cards, concept maps, and flashcards. This is material you can carry around with you and review whenever you catch a break. My favorite is the pocket guides. You can take those anywhere.

WORK WHERE YOU LEARN.

For every single diagnosis we covered, we formulated a plan that we presume will work. We also produced a list of interventions to make sure we can effectively implement our plan. Use these examples to create effective plans and interventions for every individual student diagnosis. By doing this, you are mastering how to apply the nursing process using familiar problems. If you are already in nursing school, I hope this exercise has improved your understanding of the nursing process: assessment (self, school, finances, learning and personality types) and now diagnosis and planning focused on problems student nurses face in the program. In the following chapters, we continue to follow through other parts of the nursing process.

CHAPTER 9

Clinical Rotations, Preparedness And Success

Clinical Rotations

This chapter focuses on the implementation of successful habits during a clinical setting, which should guarantee success. To implement is to do. In the clinical setting, we are doing. I introduce habits that I utilized to become successful in the clinical setting.

Primarily, do not take shortcuts; learn the right practice in the beginning and you will not have problems in the future. In my culture, we also have a saying that states, "You cannot straighten a tree that is aged. If you attempt to, you will break its back." This implies that it is easier to straighten a leaning tree while the stem is young. If you attempt to do it much later, you can break its back. Same goes for years of wrong practice. It is harder to fix what is already broken. From the beginning, endeavor to practice the right way.

I remember the excitement when I received my nursing school uniform and stethoscope. I was so proud. I took several pictures and posted them on my social media accounts. I even had a name for my stethoscope.

My first clinical was at Tufts Medical Center in Boston. A substantial experience I must say. I will always be grateful for my first clinical instructor. She built my confidence and taught me how to be a great nurse. My fondest memory of her lessons was when she walked my clinical group and I into a room. She then asked us what was missing. As a nursing student, you tend to rush to clinical reasoning as opposed to the environment. She then proceeded to educate us about a therapeutic environment and Florence Nightingale's theorem. Her emphasis on a healing environment made me become a better nurse. When I walk into a patient's room, I quickly scanned the environment for safety and healing promotion.

When you walk into a room, make sure to let in the light, position a patient's chair by the window so they could view the scenery, take the urinal off the table, and clear clutter. You do not want a food tray to be placed on a dirty table.

Pay attention to details such as preferences of diverse populations. People of Asian origin often prefer taking pills with warm water. Tufts Medical Center serves a lot of people of Asian origin. I learned that many people of Asian origin viewed disease in two categories, warm and cold. They also used different therapies to treat the diseases. If a disease is believed to be caused by heat, the therapy is cold treatment and vice versa. Review Yin and Yang in the context of health to further understand this concept.

My instructor embodied holistic nursing care in every sense. Your first clinical instructor can really break or make your nursing career. I am glad I had a great first experience. Some students do not have this opportunity to be inspired by great nurses. If you find yourself in a situation where your instructor makes it hard for you to learn, follow protocol and hierarchy and see to it that you have a positive experience because this can impact your career and nursing practice.

Preparing for Clinical (rules and regulations)

Read your school clinical expectations manual. It is imperative that you know what you can and cannot do as a student nurse. There are nurses who will always think that they are helping you out by letting you do some things that you should not, but eventually, this could get you in trouble.

If you are not sure about being able to do something, make sure to let them know politely that you are not competent, and would prefer to observe. You must protect yourself, your patients, and your academic institution. Reading the manual will clearly spell out the activities you are not allowed to do. Also, listen to your clinical instructor and professors.

Student nurses are accountable for their actions in a clinical setting. There is a misconception that you are practicing under the license of your instructor. The Nurse Practice Act in your state has a clause that applies to your state. Do well to become familiar with it, and practice within your scope. This is a habit you should adopt. Always refer to the Nurse Act, and work place policies to protect yourself and the patient. As a student nurse, the schools you attend stipulate how you practice with reference to the Nurse Act in your state and the organization where you have clinical rotations.

Once you question anything in the clinical setting, your resources are:

- Your academic institution.
- The organization to which you are assigned. Note that organizations vary in policy. Refer to policies unique to those organizations. Know where to find these polices. On the first day of orientation, ask your instructor to show you where you can find the organization's policies.
- Your clinical instructor.
- Review the Nurse Act in your state. Pay close attention to the student nurse clause.

While in the clinical setting, you are responsible for your own practice. You are NOT, practicing under your clinical instructor's license. Should you proceed to make a decision that results in the loss of life or injury, you will be held responsible especially if you bypassed the policies that would have prevented the incident.

How to Excel in your Clinical Rotations

Be prepared. The clinical usually aligns with classroom content. Review content that concerns the clinical floor that you are placed on. I was assigned to a step-down cardiac surgery unit for both professional nursing and medical-surgical rotations. Preparation meant reviewing cardiac medications, adverse drug reactions and nurse interventions, and cardiac care plans and implications. Knowing the general care of post-cardiac surgery patients, and what nursing diagnosis to expect from these patients was very vital in my success during this rotation.

In your first clinical rotation, you learn who a professional nurse is. As mentioned earlier, nursing is a profession of relationships— relationships with our patients, work colleagues, and the organizations that we work for. The most important of these relationships is the one we form with the patient. For nurses to intervene and impact a patient's life, they should have formed a therapeutic working relationship. Learning how to communicate effectively and respectfully will enable you to succeed in the clinical setting. Nursing is also a multi-disciplinary relationship that relies on the same concepts to achieve excellent clinical outcomes.

Who is a professional nurse?

- Always presents self in a professional manner. Adheres to dress code, and always wears a badge for easy identification.

- A professional nurse should be on time for assigned work shifts.
- Communicates effectively and efficiently. You should try something like incorporating an introduction that works for you such as; Good morning Mr. Doe, my name is Sandrah, and I will be your nurse from this time to this time. Then proceed to warm your way into the conversation. My instructor always cautioned us against introducing ourselves while updating the white boards. Face the patient when you introduce yourself.
- Effective communication is required when you pass on the nursing report, update a team member or family, and so on.
- Abides by the organization's work policies and those of the state in which they practice.
- Abides by the nursing code of ethics

Review this information repeatedly and form a foundation for yourself that is based on professionalism. Remember, we form all our habits in the beginning.

SBAR communication tool

A student nurse will learn earlier on to communicate with efficiency. This tool appears challenging to begin with but practice it by using everyday scenarios that will improve the efficient and results-oriented application.

Example 1:

I am having an unkempt hair day. I cannot wear my hair to work today. This is the situation.

Background: I trimmed my hair a few months ago. The length is unmanageable. I wear knots overnight to grow it out again.

Assessment: Hair is in knots. The knots are not neat; therefore, I cannot wear them to work. The hair appears shabby, unkempt, and dry. It does feel dry when I rub my hands through it.

Recommendation: Undo the knots, condition, and shampoo the hair, and comb it out. Perhaps consider a trim to even out the hair.

I have used an everyday situation to explain SBAR communication. Use simple regular situations and develop an SBAR. Once you have understood this concept, apply it to the patients you are assigned to on your next rotation. This is the tool you will use to communicate with other health care workers and to document.

Example 2:

You have been assigned a patient that has a Foley catheter. The nursing aide walks up to you and says, "The patient is acting funny; this is not like them." Once you walk into the room, you assess the patient's mentation. Mr. Doe knew where he was when you came in earlier. Now he thinks he is at home and he is looking for his wife. His wife passed a while ago.

Situation: The patient appears confused. He does not seem to know where he is, and he is looking for his wife. Or, there is a noticeable change in patient's mentation.

Background: 89-year-old male with a history of CVA, neurogenic bladder with a chronic Foley (List only the history that applies to the situation stated). He presented to the hospital with a temperature of 100.4 despite taking Tylenol.

*Assessment: Assess mentation (Is this usual?), vital signs, urine output (color, odor). Check prior lab results and list anything that pertains to what you are suspecting. *Assessment is a collection of pertinent data that supports the situation and is referenced in the patient's background.

*Recommendation: Page MD, collect urine sample. Place on fall precautions (bed and chair alarm, fall risk band and soaks) for safety given mentation change.

*the recommendations are your interventions as a nurse. This is where you integrate risk reduction, safety, and health promotion measures. In simple terms, how you make the situation better.

You will implement nursing interventions to ensure safety while you wait for orders. To implement nursing diagnosis, you must understand nursing diagnosis.

Every patient is at risk for falls and infection given the hospital setting. There are multiple nursing diagnoses. To broaden your scope of nursing diagnosis, start practicing more complex diagnosis. While in the clinical setting, create five nursing diagnoses for the patients you are assigned to. Remember to place the diagnoses in the order of priority.

This I know will make you better at formulating a nursing diagnosis. A nurse's actions are only as good as their diagnoses. Nursing diagnosis will guide care and ensure that the patient's immediate needs are met as well as help progress the patient toward long-term goals. I also purchased a small nursing diagnosis book I referenced in the clinical setting.

Always Be Prepared.

Preparation places you ahead of the learning curve. Instead of wasting time looking up content during clinical, you should absorb more content and focus on application of knowledge in the clinical setting.

My pediatrics clinical instructor gave us the patient's diagnosis the evening before the assignment. This does not violate HIPPA. All we knew was the diagnosis. The diagnosis identified rare chronic conditions that required us to review prior to the day of the clinical.

I worked at a chronic long-term pediatric facility, and the patient population was the same throughout the clinical rotation. All we knew was the diagnosis, not the patient's specifics like their names, date of birth and so on. Knowing the diagnosis, the evening before gave us ample time to look it up and put two and two together before meeting the patient. I found that I was better prepared in this clinical. This was only possible because this facility was rehabilitative. The turnover of patients in an acute medical surgical setting does not permit the use of this technique (knowing a patient's diagnoses prior to the clinical).

I personally believe that student nurses would benefit from working in rehabilitation and nursing home facilities because the pace is slower and allows for learning to take place.

Always inquire

Ask questions. Whether they are stupid or not, ask anyway. Your instructor is there to teach you and will appreciate your interest. Do not ask common sense questions such as when a patient admitted when you can simply look it up. I have found that it irritates people.

"You know what you know, and you do not know what you do not." Anonymous

I would rather I look like a fool rather than make a detrimental mistake that could place my patient in imminent danger. Another good practice to adopt is writing down the questions and doing some research about your questions before asking.

You Are the Company You Keep.

Partner with equally enthusiastic students. Working with a stronger student will make you stronger yourself. Some students are very gifted and can accomplish tasks at a higher level. These are the students you want to have in your circle. Make friends with them. There are couple of people that get through nursing school because of such partnerships. With time, you will realize that you learn from each other. Never work alone. It is dangerous especially for a novice in a clinical setting. The fact is that everything is new to you unless of course, you were a nurse in your past life, which is very unlikely. Working alone will put you at risk of making mistakes. You do not know it all. No one does in nursing school or even in practice. In this profession, we are always learning. Refer to the chapter that explores nurseships to reiterate why choosing the right friends is important.

Time Management

Arrive early, have a good and heavy breakfast. You barely know when your break is, and you want that mind to stay razor sharp. Another thing to do before clinical is to have a good night's sleep the night prior to clinical. Doing all this sounds like a no brainer but doing these things will enhance learning. Pack your bag the day before, placing things like pieces of paper, stethoscope, and a pen or pencil in your uniform pockets. I write a lot. I would take notes from my clinical day and review them after clinical and reflect on the things I still need to learn. Buy a clipboard; it is beneficial.

Knowing the Expectations

Every clinical is different, and so are the expectations. My fundamentals and acute or medical surgical clinical were geared toward professionalism, competency in SBAR, and nursing diagnosis.

In my maternity clinical, we focused on maternal physiological changes during all trimesters and postpartum complications. Know the medications neonates receive when and where, the newborn assessments and complications of birth, post-partum care and complications, and a lot of anticipatory guidance.

The objective of the maternity clinical is to learn how to educate the new mother, preparing the mother for the child's growth and so on and so forth. Your nursing instructors are very observant and will point out where you are lacking.

Nursing school lays a foundation, and with every tier, you have higher expectations that involve prior objectives. You must meet prior competencies to be extremely successful in your next tier. A good rule of thumb is to find out the objectives of each clinical rotation. At the end of the rotation, assess yourself and determine your level of competency.

A successful student nurse will:

- Know the objectives of the clinical rotation.
- Save their clinical instructor's phone number and email.
- Read their school's clinical expectations and never perform any activity they are not sure of.
- Prepare ahead of the clinical. You know the floor you are assigned to by now. Know the popular medications, drug reactions, and nursing interventions and implications.
- Ask questions. Better safe than sorry.
- Arrive on time, have a good breakfast and rest well the night off.

One is always better safe than sorry. Practice by state nurse act in your state, school and organization polices. In the next section, I focus entirely on the practicum. The practicum is the final clinical setting. In this final clinical setting, we are expected to have built a foundation of professionalism. In this section, I continue to introduce habits that enabled me to be successful in the clinical setting.

The Practicum

A senior practicum is your final clinical setting in nursing school. Many schools will try to accommodate students and place them in areas they are interested in. The expectations of your senior practicum are different from those of regular clinicals. In this section, I speak of my experience and the impact it had on my learning. You will be surprised at how much you know at the end. I wrote the practicum portion in real time. I started writing before the practicum, during the Winter break of 2017. The following events are in real time.

***

I have an introductory preceptorship meeting in the first week of January. I am both excited and looking forward to working very closely with my preceptor to sharpen my nursing skills. Like the start of any clinical rotation, class, or simulation, I find out what the objectives are. The objectives are the school's expectations. I then evaluate myself and determine what my expectations are too. My expectations are to practice independently as a student nurse and then as a novice in the clinical setting with little to no assistance.

Always sent your own expectations. Using the nursing process, access your needs and devise a plan that will enable you to meet these expectations.

This semester, I plan to utilize the simulation lab and practice all the skills one at a time, starting with the fundamental skills and working myself up to complex care. I needed to review fundamental skills because it has been a long time since I performed them. I want to feel confident when I graduate. This is my last semester in nursing school.

I mapped out a successful semester before I resumed school. I would evaluate my needs based on the previous semester and determine what I needed to work on the following semester. This habit enabled me to start the following semester with clarity.

On January 2, 2017, I found out that I had been placed on the Cardiac Thoracic Intensive Care Unit for my preceptorship. Yes, I am overjoyed and nervous at the same time. As previously mentioned, I have taken a specific liking to cardiology, and I was hoping for an ICU placement and I am so glad I ended up with this placement.

A lot of preparation for my preceptorship mirrors that of the regular clinical. The preceptorship, however, is on another level because I am paired with one nurse. Today I begin my preparation by noting my preceptor's name and email number just like I have done in the past. I will contact my preceptor a week or so prior to the day of orientation and introduce myself.

I already have my work, and work schedules figured out for this quarter. This is important because unlike regular clinical, I have clinical only on the days my preceptor works. We were told to have completed 140 hours of self-scheduling by the end of the rotation. My professors warned us not to overload hours in the beginning but spread them throughout the semester. That is an advice I intend to allow.

I am religious, and I do not mean to force my beliefs on anyone, but prayer is an absolute necessity. I pray for my instructors at the very start of the semester. My prayer involves asking God to guide them and for them to teach me the best way they know how. My prayer request is that she welcomes me with open arms and instructs me to the best of her ability. God works in miraculous ways, and I always have relied on prayer to guide me.

You know your placement, what next?

Chances are that you too will know your placement ahead of time. Knowing what kind of floor, you are placed on before the start of the semester will give you ample time to prepare and refresh previous knowledge specific to the clinical floor and specialty. Part of my preparation was reviewing all the cardiac content including medications. During my pharmacology class, I made medication flash cards specific to systems. The cardiac stack is going to be in use this semester because again to be successful, you must go the extra mile. Part of maximizing my learning in the clinical setting is to prepare ahead of time so that the time I spend in the clinical setting involves mostly implementation (doing) of concepts, interventions, and performing skills.

Another thing one can do is find out what type of patients you will take care of on the assigned unit. This being an intensive care unit, I expect my patients to be hooked onto multiple equipment. And because this is a cardiovascular intensive care unit, I will need a refresher on all the complications that can arise from surgeries and the emergency protocol therein.

A better prepared nursing student is a great student. This enables you to utilize the time spent in the clinical setting to soak in knowledge and practice skills and not find knowledge while you should be learning. Unpreparedness is the root of anxiety in clinical settings. The stress that accompanies being overwhelmed can be prevented by being prepared. This is how I remained cool-headed when faced with multiple tasks.

Ensure that all the requirements needed are fulfilled before the start of the semester. I almost missed a clinical rotation because I held off getting a TB skin test and when I finally took the test, it was positive just a week from the start of the rotation. I needed a chest x-ray that very week. I work in a clinical setting and must have been exposed somehow. My prior TB skin tests were always negative, and I saved the test for last minute thinking that would be the case. This is the first time I really did panic, and I swore never to procrastinate again.

Staying in touch with friends over the break is particularly important as well. Staying in touch means that you will not miss any critical information. My closest friend through nursing school was excellent with requirements, and I found myself relying on her to pace myself while she relied on me as well for other things. Friends will make nursing school a much more tolerable experience.

Preceptorship Orientation Day

The instructor stressed one thing that I realized was extremely important. She repeatedly said that while in clinical practice, we should adhere to learning the good practices because they stick with us forever. Train yourself to do everything right, and by the book, and you will never lose the skills.

My preceptorship orientation instructor was awesome. Here are a few of the tips that I learned from my practicum that could be of use to you:

- Always keep the patient the center of focus. When in doubt, always ask if what you are about to do or doing is what is best for the patient. Remember, we are in an interdisciplinary field and there are a lot of resources, you are never alone. Use your resources.
- Know the policies. Look them up with your preceptor. Never do anything that is beyond your scope of practice. Whenever you are unsure, ask. Better safe than sorry.
- Your preceptor should be present during medication administration, at least for the first few times until you are

signed off for competency. During my practicum, all my medication administration was supervised given the intensity of the unit and patient.

- Arrive early. Read the off-going nurse and physician notes. Most times you will find the plan of the day in the physician notes. During rounds, you will be able to clarify the plan and goals for the day. Reviewing the care plan also enables you to focus your interventions.

- Email your preceptor and introduce yourself as soon as you find out who they are. Remember to be professional, polite, and precise while working with your preceptors and everyone else.

- Review the nurse practice act regulations that pertain to student nurses. Know the activities you can and cannot do. Students (I included) always thought that we are performing under our preceptor's license. This is not true. All students' nurses are liable for everything once in a clinical setting. This is an appropriate time to familiarize oneself with your school of nursing policy. It is during preceptorship that a nursing student is most likely to perform as an individual. Simply put CYA (Cover your ass, do everything according to provided guidelines)!

I recall being nervous about the ICU because this was a new experience and the patients were critically ill. All my prior clinical placements were on Step down and Med-Surgical floors, and I had become accustomed to the pace and patient population.

The ICU was a whole different ball game. Nevertheless, I was determined to master this animal and tame it. I wanted to be afraid. Matter of fact, I needed to be afraid. Being afraid meant that I was more cautious. These patients on the ICU are very acute. Which means that I am more likely to kill someone with one stupid mistake.

Having assessed myself, I produced a plan. My nursing diagnosis at this point was extreme stress related due to the intensity of my clinical placement. I did not let this feeling wear me down. I approached every day with a goal and a plan. At the end of every clinical day, I asked my preceptor what she thought I needed to work on. I wrote notes, revisited the notes, did my research, and made sure to apply this material the next time I went into clinical.

How to Manage Preceptorships

Scheduling

My school of nursing gave the opportunity to self-schedule our practicum hours, and schedule preceptor hours throughout the semester. Do not overwhelm yourself in the beginning by scheduling more than 12 hours in the first few weeks. Pacing yourself is also beneficial for learning purposes. Concepts are introduced as the semester goes on and if you attempt to complete your preceptor hours ahead of schedule, you miss practicing skills you learn much later in the semester.

Schedule open lab hours and practice skills more often. This is the last semester and being confident while performing skills is particularly important. Your school of nursing will have expectations to be completed with every rotation. If you notice that you are weak in an area, practice the skills in the simulation lab ahead of your clinical. This will enable you to perform skills with confidence in the clinical setting.

Planning and Problem-Solving

Identify a problem, work on getting better. My clinical faculty was very friendly and offered so many clues to get me through preceptorship. One thing I found extremely helpful was practicing the techniques as you learn them. I had a lot of trouble with the IV pumps. I went home, watched videos, and practiced on poles that were not used at my work place. The more you do, the better you get.

My clinical faculty also informed us that we should know the day's plan and times for medications. I was placed on the ICU and unfortunately never had a patient assigned to me because of the clinical nature of the patients on those floors. I shadowed the nurse and was told to be assertive with my need to learn or I would not learn much.

Have a plan for every clinical day. While reviewing for a cardiac exam, I came across an auscultation technique I had never used. I wrote that down to perform for the next clinical. Having a goal for your clinical day increases your efficacy in the clinical setting. At the end of the day, evaluate how well you did.

Using Checklists

One thing I have also learned during my preceptorship is that I should always have a checklist. You should never rely on memory to remember tasks. My checklists have boxes that I check off once the task is complete.

Ideal checklist were the brief ones. Use abbreviations that you can recall, check patient orders, and make sure that you have not missed a thing. Be sure to arrange the tasks in the order of priority. This prompted me to always arrive 30 minutes before clinical starts. I had realized that I needed time to formulate a checklist before the report. During the report, I filled in the blanks. This is something I devised halfway through my clinical hours. Had I done this sooner, I would have saved myself a lot of time.

When I gave the report the first time, I was not as confident. Having learned this, I planned to give a report every single time I went in no matter how complex, and every time I listened to the criticism, I focused on the criticism to become better. I continued to plan, to do more for competencies I felt I was weak in. I read more. I watched videos and re-evaluated myself. I utilized checklists to give reports on the ICU. I simplified my checklist to ABC.

Example of the checklist I used in the ICU

Airway	Breathing	Circulation
• Inbutated? • Ventilator settings • Last ABGs • VAP interventions • Neuro	• Ventilator settings • Medications? • Respiratory sytem • Extubation plan?	• Arterial BP • Cardiaovascular system • Cardiac medications? • ECMO? IABP? • Postop day?

The above is an example of what my checklist would look like. During report, I would reference my checklist and review the systems from head to toe giving my assessments, changes in systems and nursing interventions performed during the day.

I was my own harsh critic. The ICU is very intimidating for a new nurse, and even more intimidating for a student nurse. It is completely okay to be less confident in such a setting. Confidence will make a student more likely to make a mistake. Even when I could tell that my preceptor was irritated by me asking if it was okay for me to perform an activity, I still let her know every single time so that she was always aware of what I was doing.

***

Clinicals should be fun and allow for students to implement what they have learned in theory. I hope that my clinical experiences and lessons are a valuable resource for you. There is a lot more to explore on the subject, but the most important takeaways are that you can practice safely by following your state's nurse act, along with school and organization policies. Always think safety and risk reduction in the clinical setting. Use checklists to enable you to prioritize and when not sure, ASK.

CHAPTER 10

Test-Taking Strategies and Nursing Tips

Test Taking

Test-taking efficacy is the ability to comprehend and extract data ONLY pertinent to the question. To answer a question correctly, you must understand what the question implies, as well as extrapolate the important data.

I honestly think test taking is a craft one must learn. The craft involves learning to consistently to pull out the most important information. This is a learned skill. We learn by practicing. And before you master something, you fail.

There are also multiple test-taking strategies that cover one's behavior prior to, during and after the test. Sleep, for example, is necessary to function at your highest level of cognition, but I cannot deny that there have been times I walked into a test with less than three hours of sleep the previous night and still excelled. We all develop success mannerisms, and once they have worked, we tend to stick with them. I reviewed content the night before my examinations and stayed up late.

I prepared for tests by taking tests prior to exam day. How else do you head to a battlefield without trying out your weapon? I made sure to spend the last two days prior to exams testing myself NOT reviewing content. Yes, I would do up to at least 200 questions and read the rationales for every question—even for the questions I had right. This habit helped me understand why I was choosing certain answers, and the mechanism/rationales behind my choices.

I made myself familiar with priority questions by testing myself on priority questions frequently. This enabled me to identify the nature of the question before answering. When you notice that a question is a priority question, apply different priorities starting with ABCs. Your first choice in most cases will be an answer that maintains the airway. If you have two answer options such as elevate the bed and apply supplementary oxygen, raising the head of the bed is the right answer because if it is not an emergency, you always want to perform the least invasive intervention. If it is an emergency, such as burn patient with stridor, your interventions are going to be to intubate because delay would compromise the airway and lead to loss of life.

Here is a list of priorities and test applications:

- Airway, breathing circulation (blood pressure, heart rate, pulse, etc.): A patient with stridor (airway emergency) takes priority over a patient with low blood pressure.

138

- Vital signs. Taking vital signs is an initial assessment. Checking the oxygen saturation of a patient that is short of breath comes before placing them on oxygen. You always want to know what the patient's oxygen saturation is before applying oxygen. A patient might simply be anxious and will need different interventions in that scenario. Always assess before planning or implementation/act. Therefore, assessing vital signs is a priority.

- Maslow's hierarchy of needs. You have a confused elderly man with a history of falling and a patient that is hysterical because they have just received an unexpected diagnosis. The patient that will require first response is the elderly man who might be at risk of falling if not attended to. Safety takes priority. Think safety and risk reduction when presented with similar questions.

- Emergent versus non-emergent. You have two patients that have been in an accident. One has a compound fracture of the fibula and is alert and oriented with stable vital signs and the other patient has a femur fracture and is currently alert and oriented with a blood pressure of 92/50. The latter is emergent and takes priority over the patient with a compound fracture. Fractures of the femur can result in deadly complications that lead to loss of life. Think complications and minimize risks.

- Acute versus chronic. A patient with pneumonia and saturation of 88% takes priority over a COPD patient with expiratory wheezing and saturation of 88% on room air. Both are airway conditions; however, the latter is a chronic condition, and the body has adjusted to that level of oxygen. Expiratory wheezing indicates an exacerbation of the COPD that can be managed with steroids and nebulizer treatments. Pneumonia on the other hand is an acute illness that requires immediate intervention because it can progress to sepsis or bacteremia if the response is delayed. Both are airway/breathing patients, but one presents with an acute condition and the other a chronic condition.

- Noninvasive before invasive. Before you put oxygen on a patient that is short of breath with low saturation, elevate the head of the bed, and check function of equipment. If these interventions do not rectify the problem, apply oxygen.

Priority questions are usually the most challenging. Once you understand priorities, you become competent at test taking. Invest time in learning the priority concepts by taking lots of priority questions until you understand how these questions are posed.

Multiple Choice Questions

The only way to become good at multiple questions and choosing the right answer is by answering a lot of questions and reading the rationales. When testing oneself, read the rationales for both the questions you have right and wrong to understand better why the answer was wrong or right.

The more you know about a topic, the easier it is for you to eliminate the wrong options. Multiple questions are a bunch of true or false options. Read the answer and decide if it is true or false. Eliminate the false options as you go.

Use the true or false strategy for multiple test questions

I found that doing concept maps helped me to know ONLY what was important to know. When answering multiple questions, you are simply eliminating an option that does not apply to the topic in question.

Do not re-read multiple questions, once you answer the question, move on. Otherwise, you are forced to select options you did not consider earlier because you are now second guessing yourself.

Again, practice makes perfect. If you are weak in multiple choice testing, test yourself more.

Calculations

Practice makes perfect. Unfortunately, I have no tricks to trade off. If you are weak in mathematics, consider getting a tutor and utilize question banks. Perform as many calculations as you can.

Master adult medical surgical class and conquer pediatric medical surgical.

Adult med-surgical and child care nursing are extremely broad. Once you master adult med-surgical, pediatric med-surgical is a breeze with only a few changes in some systems. The changes are mostly with congenital diseases and developmental level interventions.

First, you are tasked to understand the systems. Therefore, anatomy and physiology are foundational for both adult and pediatric med-surg. Build a solid foundation. Succeeding in nursing school really depends on one's foundation.

After you have understood the systems and how they normally function, you will recognize the signs and symptoms when these systems begin to fail. Using prior pathophysiology and microbiology classes, you will note how a failed system affects the individual and the systems.

What you see is signs and symptoms of system failure, and medical surgical nursing shows you how you should intervene. Your nursing interventions will assist you in optimizing and maintaining health despite system failure.

There are multiple systems. The only way to condense this knowledge is to utilize concept maps. Concept maps will make it easier to understand conditions and save a lot of time during review. They take time to create, but they are a resource beyond nursing school. My concept maps were so well created, I used them to review for the NCLEX.

These are the signs and symptoms you will include in a concept map:

- When one sees red currant jelly stool, what gastrointestinal condition do you suspect? This is indicative of a specific gastrointestinal condition. The stool is red because there is blood and it is jelly like because the intestinal tract has mucus. The condition is intussusception. To alienate this condition from multiple GI conditions that have the usual signs and symptoms (nausea, vomiting, diarrhea, anorexia, etc.), identify what makes the condition unique so you can perform interventions specific to the condition in question. Note that there are interventions unique to this condition. When you have a test question that gives you signs and symptoms, you will able to select the correct answer/intervention because you know the medical diagnosis.

Concept Map of Intussusception

Intussusception (Definition)			
Risk factors Risk population	Signs and symptoms/ presentation	Diagnostics and labs	Nursing intervention
	***Red currant jelly like stool ***bile stained emesis	Ultrasound, X-ray	List interventions in order of priority. Listing the interventions in order of priority will enable you to select the best option on tests when approached with questions on Intussusception
	Fever, severe abdominal pain, n/v/d		

***If you are a visual learner, you can attach a diagram to your map or a link to YouTube that explains the condition.

- A question mentions that your patient has a red butterfly facial rash? You are given a list of interventions. First you need to know what condition causes this specific rash in order to select the right answer. This condition is systemic lupus erythematous. If you are not able to identify this condition, you will not be unable to choose the right option. Use the concept map example above to create a concept map.

- You palpate an olive-green mass in the upper abdomen, rigid board abdomen. What is the condition?

The above are classic signs and symptoms that are unique to the disease processes they accompany. Your signs and symptoms or client presentation are part of what the concept map will highlight "classical clinical signs and symptoms." Do not waste your time writing expected signs and symptoms such as nausea, emesis, and diarrhea. Focus on what makes that condition unique. Creating concept maps will help you filter out what is important to know. Refer to the chapter on concept maps to learn how to concept map with efficacy.

FOCUS ON THE UNIQUENESS OF THE DISEASE PROCESS AND CONDITION

The exclusivity of maternity (mother and baby)

Everyone thinks that assessing mother and baby is easy. I beg to differ. You have two patients here, mother and baby. You are monitoring how the mother affects the baby's condition or how a baby's change in status can affect the mother at the same time.

Maternity is incredibly unique and has a lot of terms that are specific to this population. There are terms such as Nadele's rule, station, gestation age, APGAR scoring, etc. Knowing the emergent and non-emergent conditions is a key area of focus, as you will quickly learn how to eliminate what is not a key area.

For example, a seven-month pregnant woman whose water broke 24 hours ago is more emergent than a nine-month pregnant woman whose water just broke. The former is at a higher risk of complications such as, premature neonatal distress and infection and that needs immediate intervention. Between the two client presentations, always ask yourself the question, "Which client complications will I have if I do not respond immediately?" The next question would be, "What complications are deadly? That is, will it result in death, injury, or harm?" These questions will always sieve through available options and help you to focus your answers.

There are also priority questions that will require you to choose between mother and baby. Here is when you will apply priorities and determine who is more stable.

The Use of Acronyms

Produce acronyms for processes, stages, values, etc. There are acronyms for remembering cranial nerves, medications, client presentations, EKG rhythms, and disease presentations. I found that the acronyms I formulated on my own stood the test of time. Michael Linares on YouTube has some of the most fun ways to recall information too. There are always new and exciting ways to retain and/or recall information.

Before testing, I would write down acronyms that were expected to be on tests. I also wrote down general guidelines to guide my testing. I used priority setting (ABCs, vital signs, change in mental status), nursing process, emergent versus non-urgent, physiological versus psychological, and safety. I would do this before beginning the exam. This habit always helped me start test questions at ease.

Acronyms save time and enable one to recall complex information and processes.

Nursing Tips

How to Use your Assigned Textbook

Knowing how to use the text to your benefit saves you time. You do not need to read the whole text to pass. You need to know how to find what you need immediately.

Instructors in my college had the syllabus available for review before school started and having your book in time will enable you to begin pacing yourself. You do not want to find out too late that you could have maximized the text to excel in the class. Start by browsing the book and looking at how the chapter is set up. This helps you know where to find information with ease. An example is knowing where to find the definition, the stem or vital information, and as you progress, you will begin to realize that the last paragraph is usually the recommendations. Nursing books are pretty much organized the same.

I learned that chapters were set up in the SBAR format. In the first paragraph, there was usually a situation or scenario followed by a definition then a history or background. Browsing the entire text and knowing where the root of the information is will help you simplify the text for future use. If you can figure out how one chapter is set up, you pretty much can pull content from other chapters with ease.

Knowing how to use your textbook also saves you a lot of time because you cannot read an entire 1000-page textbook. You simply do not have the time and you will not remember a lot of the information anyway. Unless of course, you have an incredible photographic memory.

Another efficient practice is to compare the objectives at the beginning of each chapter to those required from your instructors. PowerPoint presentations usually have objectives for the information being taught if your instructor makes those available to you.

When reviewing the text later, the objectives are your cheat sheet. This is what you NEED to know. Know the responses to the objectives. Take all the tests at the end of the chapters and review the critical thinking questions because testing yourself sharpens your understanding of the content. It sounds like a lot of work but once you have done this three times, it becomes easy. The highlighted information along with the diagrams and connotations are also important to pay attention to.

This practice will help you get the most out of the book without using the whole book. Some books also have codes that enable you to have online access to visuals. A visual learner will benefit from this tool. Some processes such as types of casts, use of walkers, and procedures might have illustrations that are easier to recall if one is a visual learner.

How to Study

Using textbooks to study is very student specific. Some students love to highlight word for word, others write in the book and use bookmarks, and some do not do anything. Practice all the ways there are and find the most efficient way that enables you to grasp information with ease. The goal is to be an efficient textbook user to save you time. At all times, remember that time is of the essence, and you must utilize it wisely.

How to Effectively Read a Textbook

Have you seen these nursing textbooks? They are HUGE! Well, I never read more than 40 pages combined. Pulling the need to know and the good to know information will not only make you an effective reader but it will save you time and sometimes money.

The instructor assigns book chapters for a class. At times, I had 7 different chapters assigned in different courses. And the due date was one week away. I had to learn to read texts and extrapolate crucial data in less than an hour for each chapter.

How to Review a Text Book

1. Read PowerPoint objectives. These objectives are your need to know. Read the PowerPoint and highlight the items that answer the objectives.

2. Compare PowerPoint objectives to the textbook objectives. Chapter objectives are located at the beginning of the chapter. This is what you need to know by the end of the chapter. With the book handy, attempt to answer the objectives by browsing the book for answers to ONLY these objectives. How? Identify the key words. If the objective states, "to understand the professional nursing model," browse the text for "professional nursing model" and review the paragraph.

3. Read the introductions, subtexts and all bold fields including viewing the images and reading the captions. Those captions under illustrations summarize content. Pay close attention to the QSEN (Quality and Safety Education for Nurses) symbols and make sure to read the highlights.

4. After you have answered all the objectives, attempt to answer the questions at the end of the chapter. Should you find that you have been asked a specific term that you could have missed, locate where the term is mentioned in the chapter and review that content. You can locate terms using the books index.

5. Always, ALWAYS test yourself after reviewing material. The more questions you answer, the better you understand the

content because not only do you learn how to think like the examiner, you learn what you need to know.

6. Always have a question bank. If you are short of money and must choose between buying a question bank instead of the textbook, buy the question bank. A question bank is what will sharpen your brain. You could read content all day, but if you cannot apply it, it is useless.

7. Buying texts brand new has its benefits. Many texts have CDs and codes that have links to websites with questions. Here is where paying a hefty price for a book benefits you. Like I said, knowing how to answer questions will teach you the priorities.

8. After you have reviewed the text, review the PowerPoints again and answer the PowerPoint objectives. It is advisable to stay ahead of the instructor. This will enable you to understand the material better during lectures.

Nursing Classes

All your classes are relevant to nursing school. Each class prepares you for success. Anatomy, physiology, pathophysiology, sociology, religion, ethics, and math and statistics are all important. Pay attention and apply the same effort in every one of your classes and ease your way through to the next class.

Your anatomy and physiology class is your key to nursing school. That followed by pathophysiology. First, you learn about the normal functions of the human body, then how the disease affects function and then, only then, does nursing begin because nursing alleviates and maintains optimum health. If everyone was healthy, we really would never need health care or nursing.

Every class lays a foundation. Take every one of them seriously because you will see this information again. I will briefly explain why every class that is in this curriculum cements your knowledge in nursing and addresses all the cores in the Code of Ethics. A lot of times students wonder why certain classes' pre-requisites are required before consideration into nursing school. My advice to you is commit yourself to these classes. Whatever you learn, you will see again. If not in school, you will encounter it in practice.

Anatomy, Physiology and Pathophysiology

The most important classes nursing students are to master are anatomy, physiology, and pathophysiology. I cannot stress the importance of leaving these classes competent. You can cram your way through and pass the classes, but it is important that you understand the concepts. The anatomy class will teach you the structure, location, and normal function of an organ or system.

Example:

Patient 1 presents with shortness of breath, dyspnea on exertion, fatigue, and reports of pink frothy sputum.

Patient 2 presents with shortness of breath, dyspnea on exertion, fatigue, enlarged liver and generalized edema.

The assessment.

These patients are similar, but their symptoms are specific to the system that is affected.

Pulling it together.

During your anatomy class, you learned that the right side carries de-oxygenated blood and the left carries oxygenated blood. You also learned that all arteries carry oxygenated blood except for the pulmonary artery and all veins carry de-oxygenated blood except for the pulmonary vein. Why is this important to know?

The two patients in the scenario all have signs of a failing cardiopulmonary system. Why is the difference important?

The side effects of the right side and the left are different because of the function of both sides. The differences in presentation determine the nursing interventions and course of treatment.

As you advance, you will add hemodynamics to the picture. You will not be able to piece information together if your knowledge is not solid. The nursing curriculum is designed to slowly introduce you to concepts one at a time, and you should be able to master the previous information to make sense of the next.

After anatomy and physiology, you will take pathophysiology. It is one of the most important prerequisites for nursing school. Pay attention to this class. This class will make or break you. You do not want to simply pass this class. You want to leave this class noticeably confident because it is the key to the nursing school puzzle. Nursing begins with pathophysiology. If you do not know how disease affects the body, how are you going to know what abnormal signs to look out for or how to intervene? Anatomy and physiology will teach you the normal signs and function of a body part and/or system. It is in pathophysiology that you will learn to tell when shit hits the fan. And as the awesome nurse you are about to be, you will intervene to halt further damage or maintain health.

Now that I have completed nursing school, I could compare the nursing curriculum to building a house. Having been an ardent reader even in my younger years. I recall the tale of the three pigs that built houses made of hay, sticks and rocks. Two houses collapsed because their foundations were not strong enough to withstand the storm and wind. The house that withstood all weather conditions had a strong foundation. One's foundation is especially important and your dedication at the start will help you sail through nursing school.

Sociology

Sociology, I think, was one of my least favorite classes because it was mind provoking. I was frustrated by effects of society and structure on health. When I think of health access, affordability, and availability, I think human rights.

Learning sociology helps you relate to diverse populations and race. So how does sociology relate to nursing? How are nurses involved? Should we as nurses be bothered in the least about how humans relate and socialize? Is that not someone else's job? A social worker perhaps? The answer is no. As we know or will learn, there is a need to diversify the workforce to eradicate health disparities. This class introduces nurses to the social determinants of health such as how one's race, area code, profession, education level, household structure, etc., determines and predicts health. With this understanding, an informed nurse can implement practices with the knowledge that race can determine health outcomes as well as outreach.

Math and Statistics

Half or more of the population including myself, do not care for math or statistics. The sad truth is that these two are not going anywhere. One of the key interventions performed by nurses is giving medications. Mathematics is ESPECIALLY important. I am sure we have heard of med errors that have led to premature deaths. Practice, practice, and practice. I am no fan of math but believe me, math is doable. Do not feed into the myths.

Oh, and statistics is everywhere. You will see it in use again. Qualitative research nursing will require you to have some baseline knowledge of p-scores to correctly interpret data. Who knows, you might choose to work in research.

Ethics

As a future nurse, it is imperative that you know right from wrong. Ethics will dive into that. A nurse is expected to make ethical decisions daily and to practice this effectively. We are to learn about the several types of ethical systems and how they apply to nursing so that when we are faced with an ethical dilemma, we can problem solve using these learned models.

Religion

Another important class is religion. As nurses, we are to withhold judgement, avoid enforcing our beliefs on others and to uphold our patients' beliefs. Knowing the diverse types of religions and their expectations helps prepare us to practice genuinely. A big one is Jehovah's Witnesses who do not accept blood transfusions. Having a basic understanding of religions and expectations will enable you to advocate for your patient and intervene appropriately.

Elsevier's Evolve Platform

If you are using a textbook published by a company called Elsevier, you will have to access the Evolve website. These websites have question banks of more than 1000 questions with rationales. The

Saunders NCLEX preparation book for example has access to over 5000 questions. Nine hundreds of which were pharmacology questions.

There are also other publishers that grant access to platforms similar to Evolve. These other platforms provide similar access to test banks, image banks, videos and more.

As you have learned, test taking in nursing school is so much different from what you are accustomed to. A smart student will study, tackle questions on the subject to be tested and read rationales to find out what the questions are looking for. Reading the rationales aligns your thinking with the tester and prepares your mind so that you know what to look for in the question. This will help you select the correct answer. There is a good chance that you will see the same questions repeatedly, and the rationales will be broad enough to direct your thinking for associated questions.

Online Tools and Guides for Nurses

ATI

If a school uses ATI, download the RN Mentor from the app store. There will be times when you cannot study but instead, you can use this tool on the go. I had this app on both my phone and iPad. When I had breaks at work, on the MBTA or some free time, I would open the app and do a few questions. *Remember to read the rationales.*

157

Make sure to utilize the online videos. ATI has great voice overs that demonstrate techniques. I think ATI procedure videos were the best. A lot of them are by the book. I used ATI to review skills. Once you fail a question pertaining to a skill, you are to do two things, perform the skill repeatedly or watch the tutorials over and over until it is engraved in you. To retain the skills, make sure to perform the skill in the clinical setting. I only inserted one catheter in my whole nursing school experience. And I must add that it was in the operating room and under pressure. If I had not reviewed this technique, I would have been nervous. My clinical instructor was right there to guide me. But oh boy, my heart raced. I had reviewed the procedure so many times and got tested on the skills I learned and passed it in simulation lab. The simulation lab is not a waste of time, use it.

U-WORLD

This tool is WONDERFUL! I found out about it in my last semester of nursing. I wish I had known about it earlier. Their rationales are the best thus far. It is a study tool of sorts. It costs quite a lot, but it is worth the expense. This is a tool you cannot share with another individual because it will be difficult to assess your areas of weakness. U-World will notify you of your weak areas, and if you are sharing this tool, I am afraid the assessment will not be accurate. Knowing your areas of weakness will make you a stronger student because then, you know where you need to put emphasis. You do not have to waste time reviewing what you already know.

PUREFLOW

This is another tool I started using in the last semester of nursing school. My critical care professor introduced us to this app. I am quite sure she created this app. She created other apps as well because she was just that good at technology.

If you love concept maps, this is your study tool on the go. What is better than being eco-friendly and having less paper pile up? Nothing, I suppose. It saves paper and is as effective as a bulky book can be. Concept maps group information in a way that is easier to recall but most importantly, easy to remember. I do not know if there are any other applications like this. But again, finding what works and what works for you is what matters.

Locate this app. It is a life saver. The information is secure forever and what is so awesome about this tool is that I can make changes to it as well.

Simple Nursing channel on YouTube

Mike Linares is a smart YouTube nurse that can simplify information. I do not know how he does it, but he does. If you are a visual learner and use mnemonics to recall information, Mike is your guy. I have had people explain content in a simpler way, and others that complicate the information, hence, making it harder to recall. I believe that any student can pass nursing school. All you must do is figure out the best way to conceptualize information.

Mike has all sorts of songs, simplified videos, charts, and his pharmacology review is next to the absolute best. Subscribe to his YouTube channel and cruise through nursing school. A lot of students have complained that their instructors are not doing an excellent job explaining information. Let Mike be your unpaid instructor. He is that good. Tell him I sent you, lol.

Pocket Guides

This is me finding a shortcut. This is not a wasteful buy. I promise you these guides are genius. The information is condensed and focuses on what you really need to know. Summarized guides like these also help you to know what is important to recall. From fundamentals to critical care, there is a guide. Buy one and stick it into your pocket at clinical. Now there is an effortless way to look up information when you need it.

No one has the time to read a textbook from the introduction to the references or even glossary. These guides will show you the hot spots. The nursing hot spots. Remember, time is of the essence in nursing school so use what you have wisely.

Simulation Labs

At my practicum orientation, the orienteer made a comment that I will never forget. They said, "Learn good practice in the beginning;

it will stick around forever." This means, learn by the book and you will always practice by the book.

Yes, there are shortcuts and there are things that can be bypassed. But as a student, I implore you to learn the correct way of doing things. It is tempting to go the other route, and so is losing your license, or killing someone in the process.

Simulation lab can be a pain. You are made to do skills repeatedly until you perform them with confidence. This will pay off later in practice. You will be more confident, and should anything go wrong, you have followed the protocol and procedures, therefore, you are protected.

Continue to work hard at skills. Watch videos over and over and again until the skill becomes a reflex action. It took me forever learn how to set up a sterile field without contaminating it. The more I did it, the more it became second nature, and the better I got. *A student nurse who bypasses the required technique is on their way to being a dangerous nurse.* Do not let that be you. Practice makes perfect. Perfect your skill set.

Tutors

There are classes that will be a challenge. It is best to identify them earlier on and prepare before the start of the semester or earlier on in the semester. Identifying students that scored high in the class is also helpful. They can offer tips to help you map out the class and be better prepared.

Case Studies

You can utilize case studies to develop a nursing mindset. Case studies will teach you how to think critically and extrapolate only the need to know data from a scenario. I used Winningham's Critical Thinking Cases in Nursing text while in nursing school. This text had all types of nursing (Med surgical, pediatric, critical care nursing, etc.)

While answering case studies, read the whole text and all the questions before answering questions. I found that working backwards (starting with the last question) with case studies focused my answers because I knew what the study was looking for.

Case studies are set up in a "differential diagnosis" format. This will teach you that patient presentation can mimic other conditions and that performing multiple lab and diagnostic tests will enable you to find a root cause. This is what real nursing is.

You will also learn a life time nursing skill, giving focused patient report. When a patient presents with gastrointestinal symptoms, you will focus on GI definitive tests unless other symptoms outside of the system of presentation are affected. You will benefit a lot from case studies if you do them as group because you are able to see how different students perceive information.

There are a plethora of nursing tips and test taking strategies out there. In this chapter, I only delved into a few. Some will work for you; others will be a complete waste of your time. The most important test-taking strategy is mastering priority concepts. To become a great test taker, you should be armed with the priorities. Remember to reach out to fellow students, faculty and experienced nurses and inquire about successful tips.

A GREAT TEST TAKER HAS MASTERED PRIORITY CONCEPTS.

CHAPTER 11

Graduation and Passing the NCLEX

<hr>

Graduation Day Recap

I remember walking out of my last exam like it was yesterday. It rained that day. After the test, I had plans to grab a drink with a friend, but she cancelled. I sat in the library at a computer for about an hour or so and I thought about everything that just happened. Nursing school was over! I made it. I was graduating. I earned my bachelor's degree. What a journey! I then walked to my car in the rain listening to the most fitting song in that moment. I was listening to the *Unmaking* by Nicole Nordeman

> *The Unmaking by Nichole Nordeman*
> *This is the unmaking, beauty in the breaking,*
> *had to lose myself, to find out who you are.*
> *Before each beginning, there must be an ending.*
> *Sitting in the ravel, I can see the light....*

This song is exceptionally beautiful. In a way, it signified my journey. Nursing school did not break me. It made me. The need to succeed and progressively improve on everything is manifested in this journey. The beauty of this journey is that I discovered I have what it takes to excel both in my personal and work life if I simply put in the work. Nursing school taught me this: challenging work pays off.

I can say now that throughout both my nursing pinning and graduation ceremonies, I was in disbelief. I had attained a bachelor's degree in nursing with honors! The most significant memory is walking across that stage, wearing my cap and gown and my Sigma Theta cord. I was filled with so much gratitude.

Another beautiful memory is when we walked past our professors standing side by side serenading us while we made our way down to the graduation ceremony tent. The looks on their faces said it all; they were proud, and we were overjoyed.

I spoke at my pinning ceremony. I was too excited to even focus on my speech. The instructors at my school are still some of the absolute best and it is because of them that I will teach someday. Every student nurse deserves a professor that is passionate about nursing. I learned so much from all these individuals. I could never thank them enough.

My only two regrets was my choice of dress and not taking enough pictures outside because it rained!

We worked so hard for four years to wear our gowns for only a day or two. I feel that we should wear our gowns more often because we all sacrificed a lot to get to that point. I will not wear this gown again, but it is a constant reminder of my graduation day and achievement. I always glance at it in my wardrobe and smile.

Moments like these are worth all the demanding work. If you are just considering nursing school, I am saying to you now, it is worth it. If you are tired and weary from the demands of the program, I can assure you now that your sweat is already paid for. The end is beautiful, and so is the beginning of a most rewarding career. Keep going, stay up if you must but whatever you do, never give up. The joy you will feel that day will cleanse all the tears. Hold still, the end is more than worth it.

Enjoy your graduation festivities because once that it is over, then comes NCLEX. The national exam you must pass to be licensed to practice. In the following section I talk about how I prepared for the exam and provide advice I think is pertinent to passing on the first try.

Preparing for the NCLEX

NCLEX Test Plan

I always have said that passing the NCLEX in 75 questions starts in nursing school not after nursing school. Students that have learned to test the way NCLEX examines will require less preparation to pass the exam. In nursing school, I purchased the NCLEX Saunders RN exam book and for two years, I tested myself on NCLEX style questions.

Prior to the test, read up on the nature of the test and test plan. You can find this information on the NCLEX website. Nursing schools also tend to follow the NCLEX guidelines to prepare students to test. The test plan changes every few years. Make sure you are reviewing a current test plan. Do not however base all your testing on the plan because what if the plan changes? Train your mind to go to war no matter what you are tested on. In brief, be prepared for anything.

According to the National Council of State Boards of Nursing (NCSBN) 2019 website, the test plan includes content categories. To review the categories and percentages of questions in each category, refer to this website.

I found that studying according to the NCLEX plan was extremely helpful. To review the test plan for your year, search the Web for the National Council for the State Boards of Nursing NCLEX RN Examination plan. The content and percentage of questions is clearly stated and explained. Please note that even though you have a brief overview of the exam, the content is not limited to what is outlined. This, however, is a good start. I recommend that every potential licensure candidate reviews the percentage of questions and categories ahead of preparation.

The test plan I used at the time had the following question types: 20% on management of care; 12% on safety and infection control; 9% on health promotion and maintenance; 9% on psychosocial integrity; 9% on basic comfort and care; 15% on pharmacological and parenteral therapies; 12% of risk potential and 14% physiological adaptation (2016 NCLEX RN Test Plan).

Please note that the test plan changes every couple of years. Refer to the website for the most current information.

Some students have a bad habit of asking what percentage of certain topics is on the exam and then focus on what is said to them not knowing that the test is different for us all. Do not fall in that trap. Your peer could have been tested more on maternity because the test determined maternity was their weakness. *No one knows what is coming, so prepare for everything.*

Preparing to Test

Prior to graduation, we filled out the paper work required by the board to test. We also had to sign a good conduct form that queried our criminal background. These yes/no responses would determine whether I was eligible to practice as a registered nurse.

It is imperative that students with a criminal background determine if they qualify to test way before going through these rigorous programs. What good is it for one to navigate the program successfully only to be declined by the board of nursing. Again, preparation is key. When you know what to expect, you prepare better.

Upon graduation, we were to return to school for an ATI live review for three days, eight hours each. During the review, we covered content right from fundamentals to complex care. It was amazing to see how much we had learned. During the review, I realized that I needed a refresher on content that was covered a few years ago because NCLEX can test you on anything.

We also were assigned a virtual ATI tutor. My school used ATI to prepare us for the exam. Some schools use Kaplan, others use Hurst, NRSNG, etc. Whatever tool you use, you should have been introduced to it prior to your final year.

The tutor reviewed all topics from fundamentals to critical care and determined one's readiness to pass. Once the tutor determined that you were ready, you would get a green light and then be able to pick up your testing requirements. The green light indicated that you were ready to test and pass the exam on first attempt.

As mentioned earlier, my process was going to be longer than the rest because I had a tuition balance that had to be cleared before I could even take the test. Much as I wanted to test sooner, I was not able to.

I used NCLEX Saunders, UWorld and ATI to prepare for the exam. I only used ATI to earn authorization to test. It was a school requirement. I never liked ATI because ATI is vague. The rationales are also not that helpful in understanding why the question is structured the way it is.

I could swear by both NCLEX Saunders and UWorld. These two combined will prepare you to excel if you start using them sooner. Like I mentioned, I started using NCLEX Saunders in my sophomore year and purchased UWorld in my senior year of nursing school. I took my first assessments for both UWorld and NCLEX Saunders in nursing school. The assessments revealed that I was already ready to test.

How to Use the NCLEX Saunders Elsevier Book

This is the best money you will ever spend in nursing school. This book is equipped with the right content. Purchase the book and begin using it in your sophomore year of nursing school.

- Buy the book brand new. It has a code with access to over 5000 nursing questions.
- Create an Elsevier account and enter your code. Here you will find questions on priority testing, health promotion, safety, and risk reduction.
- You will also have questions on body systems as well as content areas such as maternity and child health, fundamentals and much more.
- In nursing school, I completed about 100 questions from content areas we were focusing on at the time. The rationales

are also extraordinarily rich in knowledge. Read all the rationales and use them as study tools.

- Prior to taking the NCLEX, take the assessment, which is 75 questions. The assessment will then give you a breakdown of your strengths and weakness and you can even form a study plan focused on your weaknesses. For example, if you find that you have scored below 60% in maternity physiological changes and adaptations, your plan should be to review physiological changes and adaptations and then test more in this category until you understand how to approach comparable questions.

Purchase this book sooner and you will excel both in nursing school and the NCLEX.

How to Use UWORLD

UWORLD is a question bank with close to 2000 questions on all areas of nursing. Before beginning testing, take Test 1 without using any outside material. After the test, assess both your strengths and weakness using the graph provided. The graph will provide an accurate description of all areas including your position on the percentile curve. Test 1 will also give you a probability of either passing or failing the exam. This is your study rubric.

After Test 1, I had a remarkably high probability of passing. Every day, I did 150 questions and reviewed the rationales. I downloaded the application to my phone, and I would do questions on the go. The number of questions you do will depend on how much time you have available in the day. I worked two jobs and would take questions in groups of 30, 40 or 50. Breaking the questions into groups helped me feel less overwhelmed and yet meet my set requirements for the day.

After each test, I would look at the graphs and determine which area I was either below average or had not been tested on. The next set of questions I would choose would depend on this assessment. You must constantly evaluate one's self.

While using question banks, it is particularly important to be completely honest with yourself. Do not use any outside material. The idea is that you learn to think on your own and the more you test, the better you get at answering these questions.

I found that using UWORLD exposed me to a wealth of material some of which I was not exposed to in nursing school. By adding the tutor feature on all the tests, I was able to review and enrich my knowledge base. The tutor feature is a virtual tutor that explains terms further. The diagrams and illustrations on UWORLD were splendid as well. I am a visual learner and love articulate illustrations.

The tools I used in the last two weeks were the ATI text to look up detailed descriptions and UWORLD. When I purchased UWORLD, I had 1900 questions in all areas. Starting with nursing care of the child, I tested on about 500 questions on all pediatric systems. While testing, I would read the rationales to all questions including those questions that I had correct to understand why they were the right or wrong choices. Yes, you must read rationales on the questions you fail as well to understand why your choice was wrong.

At the end of the two-week period, I had completed 80 tests ranging from 30 to 100 questions and I had covered 1800 questions. Besides UWORLD and the comprehensive ATI text, I never used any other outside material. Limiting the material, you use is also an aspect to consider. For example, the laboratory value ranges in ATI and UWORLD were different. To avoid any confusion, I familiarized myself with the UWORLD laboratory ranges. Do not be too rigid with these laboratory tests. An abnormal lab result is evident because a level that high or low can be detrimental to human survival. Levels that are slightly off do not alter systemic function.

After completing questions in all test areas, I did Test 2 with no outside help or materials. The percentage at this point had increased and I was still placed in the "Very high" probability of passing category. I then re-assessed the graph to find out in which areas was I below average and thankfully, this time, I was above average in all areas. At this point I felt that I was ready to test. This was the week before my test date.

Review

I planned to review at least weekly. My plan was to test in August. So, I created a schedule to keep me on track. Schedules are a life saver. Here is a snapshot of what my schedule looked like:

Day of the Week	Focus
Monday	ATI content and test
Tuesday	ATI review of test and rationales
Wednesday	UWorld 100 questions with rationales
Thursday	UWorld 100 questions with rationales
Friday	UWorld 100 questions with rationales

My weekly goal was to complete at least 300 questions from either Elsevier/Saunders or UWorld but with time, UWorld seemed like the most appropriate resource. My advice is that you limit the review resources you use to avoid confusion. Find one that works and stick to it. All texts have different presentations. I used only two resources. On Saturday and Sunday, I rested. I did this for a whole month and then I was ready to test. I tested and passed the exam in 75 questions on my first attempt.

Focusing on Areas of Weakness

For fundamentals for example; I created a study plan where I would focus on safety and infection control because I found that I was weaker in that area. UWorld and Evolve will let you know what your weaknesses are. I reviewed modules and took test questions related to this area until I felt confident with my responses. Once you understand the responses a specific area looks for, you can then apply that to various nursing topics.

When doing remedial tests, ALWAYS note the areas of weakness and do more questions in that area while reading the rationales. You will find that the more you test, the more you begin to rationalize the same way as the NCLEX. You will approach related questions with ease, and you will also be able to identify the type of question before answering. I can tell that a question is looking for a risk reduction, safety, or physiological adaptation answer by reading it.

When Should You Take the Test?

Many licensure candidates ponder on this. The answer is when you are ready. It is not a race to the finish line. Some people test as soon as possible because they have jobs already lined up when they finish school. If that is not the case, review, study, and then test. Yes, it is better to test as soon as you graduate but that is individual based. The fact is that nursing jobs will still exist even a year from your test date. If you are licensed, you will always have a job.

Nursing school cultivates a culture of competition we should not continue to follow. It does not matter who takes the test first, how many tests you take, or how many times you took the test to pass. What matters is that you passed and are now licensed. The truth is, even those that do not make it the first time are good nurses; they just did not know how to test. For those that fail the first time, try again. *It is not you and what you know, it is the way you are testing.*

I wanted to test immediately to secure a job at the hospital I had applied to because there was a deadline. I am glad I had a work-school balance that held me up because God had even better plans for me. Nursing school is stressful, and so is the nursing profession. I personally feel that new graduate programs (residency nurse programs) should start at least four months after graduation to allow students some time off and vacation before starting a career. These programs will not even give you vacation for at least 6 months so why start immediately after nursing school? Let students have a well-deserved break before walking into the next stressful thing.

Newly licensed nurses are not eligible for vacation when they begin working because there are terms and conditions in their contracts that require a certain time commitment before even taking a much-needed break. These programs should look into nurses starting at least three months after graduation to allow students some time off.

I am big advocate for self-care. Yes, there are responsibilities but there is also you. Health is wealth. I am sure we all have heard of compassion fatigue. Take your time. Pace yourself and take care of yourself.

By the end of June, a month after graduation, my colleagues were uploading images of passing the board exam. I then felt pressured to test but I am glad I did not give in. Never give in to pressure to test when you are not ready. We tend to be influenced by other people's journeys and processes and instead of focusing on ourselves. We constantly place ourselves in competition to achieve what others have and yet, our journeys are different. I would think that this is the reason some students fail. They rush into it.

Unless you are ready, hold off on being pushed in that direction. The other deadly habit nursing students have is asking other students that have tested what topics they should expect. The NCLEX is complex. Your weakness is tested more to make sure you understand the concepts. No test is going to look the same.

NCLEX and Priority Questions

As a nurse, you are expected to make more complex decisions and even decide which patient receives care before the other. With every response, ask yourself what the potential damage would be if you do not act immediately. This is what prioritization entails. What happens if you delay action? The response that escalates to death the fastest is your priority. The expectation is that when we graduate from nursing school, we can prioritize and think critically. This is what the NCLEX tests you on; your ability to critically think and prioritize.

There are a couple of guidelines that guide priority questions, and these include but are not limited to ABCs, safety, risk for harm, emergent versus non-emergent, Maslow's hierarchy of needs, physiological versus psychological, acute versus chronic, and the nursing process (before you act, you assess unless it is an emergency such as stridor; then you will act before you assess). Refer to previous chapters to review priority testing.

Fundamentals Review Questions

For a lot of students, fundamentals is a challenging review. Fundamental nursing is the most distant information to recall having completed this course at the beginning of nursing school. This area is one where you must polish up. Some of the skills we learned in this area we practiced in clinical settings while a lot of them were not covered. Inserting intravenous lines for example is a skill we only complete after licensure but that does not mean we will not be tested on the knowledge of this skill. While reviewing this area, make sure to expose yourself to as many questions as possible. If you notice that you are consistently failing a skill, this is the time to consult with a text and review the skill in its entirety or watch a video that has the steps included. ATI has the best skills review videos.

Review skills such as NGT insertion, Foley insertion, inserting an IV line, changing a sterile dressing, setting up a sterile field, etc. You will have questions that require you to rearrange the skills and put them in order or elimination by multiple choice.

Pharmacology NCLEX Review Questions

If you worked hard during pharmacology class, this will be a breeze. *Nurses are not doctors nor are they pharmacists.* We are not required to know everything. Much as medication administration is one of our most important interventions, our only task is to deliver these medications safely utilizing all the rights of medication. What we should know is how to safely administer medications. Know the adverse drug reactions and the nursing interventions should there be an adverse reaction to the drug. You should also be familiar with what the medication is intended for and the correct route. Know your rights of administration.

There are a million medications and others are still being discovered. Today I was looking at the paper and they spoke of a new cardiac medication that will treat inflammation of the heart after a heart attack and prevent further damage. My point is, there are plenty of medications out there. I am going to give you a brief overview of how I prepared for pharmacology.

I used the NCLEX Saunders prep book. I love the NCLEX Saunders book because it highlights content pertinent to the test. This book has 900 questions on medications grouped into systems. I continually tested myself and wrote down my weak areas and it is those weak areas I reviewed repeatedly until I was content with my knowledge level.

Having a drug book handy is great especially when studying pharmacology. Davis's Drug Guide was one of my favorite drug books. Make sure to buy the most up to date version. An instructor once said, "You never forget the things you look up." I believe this statement to be true. Write down the medications that you have not heard of and look them up again.

Pay the most attention to the adverse drug reactions. What is going to kill your patient should you not respond? Things like alterations in mood, such as agitation or change in level of consciousness, signify decreased perfusion to the brain. AIRWAY complications are always a priority, as well as signs, and symptoms of drug toxicity.

The routes and administration times are also imperative. Mike Linares on YouTube has awesome visual reviews of some medications. He even raps about medications. If you are a visual learner, utilize this resource. Mike Linares reviews were a great resource during nursing school. He has a UTI and Levaquin video I have never forgotten, and I only watched it once. I was able to remember that a particular antibiotic can cause tendonitis because I watched that video. His videos are very catchy.

When you are reviewing medications, you really want to focus on the side effects unique to the medication in the same class. For example, Levaquin's adverse drug reactions include tendon rupture, tendonitis, pseudomembranous colitis, and photosensitivity. The classic side effects such as nausea, vomiting, diarrhea can be caused by over 90% of the drugs on the market. Pay attention to unique side effects.

If you know the adverse drug reactions, you should then know what to do to prevent them. You can educate the patient thoroughly enough to report the signs and symptoms. You can continuously monitor the patient for the reactions and so fourth and so on.

Use the Six Rights of Medication Administration to guide your answers. When you read the question, think about what it is asking. Is it asking about something to do with the patient? Is it asking about the route? Or is it asking about a drug to drug interaction? For example, a question can ask about the route indirectly by mentioning that a patient has an NGT and is scheduled to receive an enteric coated or extended release medication. What is your intervention as a nurse? What medications are on the "Do not crash" list?

The rights of medication are your nursing guide in pharmacology. The rights of medication will enable you to think like a nurse when it comes to medication administration. For example:

- Why is it important to know the route? Can the patient tolerate the route of administration? How can I intervene if they cannot?
- What other routes can be utilized? What disease processes affect the route of administration?
- Think about the patient in question. Can they metabolize the medication? What affects one's ability to utilize the

medication? Does your patient have liver cirrhosis for example? Are they a dialysis patient? When answering pharmacology questions, focus on what the patient in question looks like.

- With polypharmacy, drug-to-drug reactions are bound to happen. Practice thinking of the patient as part of a whole, and consider, what if a patient has a history of CHF, CKD, and diabetes mellitus? What medications are they taking? Are the medications effective together? What are the compounded side effects? A patient taking ACE inhibitors, NSAIDs and potassium sparing diuretics can have a significant increase in serum potassium.

- Some medications can mask what symptoms of a disease. For example, a beta blocker can mask some side effects of hyperglycemia.

- When self-testing with pharmacology, remember to read all rationales on the questions. You will get to review other drugs in the process. Try to write them down as opposed to highlighting. Writing down things commits them to memory.

Med-Surg

The concept maps you created will save the day. I coupled my review of questions with concept maps I had created. Med-surg is such a broad topic and includes lots of systems. I used concept maps I created during nursing school to review some of the systems.

NCLEX: The Ultimate Beast

After taking my second UWORLD assessment that predicated an extremely high probability of passing the exam, I took the test. I cannot disclose the content of the examination, but I can say that confidence plays a huge role in passing this examination. I read all the questions in their entirety and all the responses, I chose my best answer and kept going. Seventy-five questions later, I had completed the exam. The exam terminates after determining minimal competency in the areas being assessed. To find out more about the exam, the content and testing strategy, visit the NCSBN or Pearson Vue website.

Everyone talks about the NCLEX exam, but no one knows what it is until they take it. This exam ONLY tests for the *minimum* knowledge a student nurse needs to have to practice as a nurse. I hope that relieves the tension surrounding that exam. Even before I tested for the NCLEX, I knew it was doable because of the amount of preparation I completed in school.

The fear students have about this test is what makes them fail in my opinion. As I often have said, *the "N" in NCLEX is for nerves.* When you let your nerves get the best of you, you will not beat this beast. So, it is not only important to prepare for the test, but it is also important to prepare your mental self before exam day. The day of the exam, I did not break my morning routine. I did what I usually do every morning. If you are like me, breaking routine makes me anxious. I then headed out to the testing site two hours ahead of time. Give

184

yourself more than enough time. This is not the time to get stuck in traffic or have surprises.

I sat in the car and listened to calming music. One hour before the test, students started coming in. A lot of them were talking about the test, but I did not. I think talking about tests before a test makes people more anxious. I personally like to stay quiet before exams. I plugged my ears and listened to relaxing music right up until we were called in to test.

Another thing to keep in mind is that the testing centers have students from various colleges and what you are taught can differ. Do not discuss things like laboratory test parameters prior to the test. Things like this will make you nervous. You want to maintain a relaxing aura before the test.

We were given small storage places to put everything we had away. The writing pad was provided by the testing site upon request.

I sat at my assigned seat and took deep breaths before I started. I proceeded to follow instructions and start the test. Again, I stuck to what worked for me in nursing school. I wrote my priorities down and started the test as calm as I could. In an hour and a half, I was out of that room. Not once did I second guess myself or linger on a question for more than a minute. I read the question, determined what the examiner wanted to know, picked an answer, and proceeded to the next question until my screen turned blue. After the 75th question, my screen went blue, and then I had to answer 30 questions that were trial testing questions for future testing purposes. The trial questions were in a different format and I cannot discuss the details. Some students will get these extra questions to enable the examining board to prepare for future tests.

In my understanding, these extra questions are used to structure future NCLEX examinations. Not everyone is tested on these questions.

After 48 hours, I found out I had passed the examination. I cannot describe how I felt. I can only say that I am very fulfilled and could not wait to have my license and practice as a nurse. Please note that not everyone that has the exam end at 75 questions has passed the exam. Some students have failed the exam when it terminated at 75 questions. The only way to know if one has passed the exam is by using the test site tool after 48 hours.

How to Pass the Board in 75 Questions

Passing the NCLEX in 75 questions begins with the first nursing class. I have covered a lot of techniques in previous chapters that will increase your chances of passing in 75.

Passing in 75 starts on the first day of nursing school. You decide there and then how you will maneuver through nursing school and how many questions you will test for to be licensed. This means building a solid foundation in the beginning. Of course, there is always room for improvement, but why wait to improve when you can start with vigor?

Be a good student or be the best. How? Refer to my previous sections about pursuing knowledge and keeping company with other enthusiastic students. Know your weaknesses early on and dedicate a lot of time to improving them. You will know soon enough what your strongest and weakest areas are.

NCLEX has a maximum of 265 questions focused on all nursing areas. Strengthen your weakness earlier on. What you do not comprehend is what you will be tested on the most. NCLEX is a computer-generated exam. The way you are tested is like the *Hunger Games*. You will be tried at each level and success at each level gets you closer to the finish line. The strongest students and those that test well will breeze through, but the good news is, you can become one or the other. Start early.

Here Are a Few Last-Minute Exercises I Found Helpful:

1. Relax. A little anxiety is productive, too much anxiety is detrimental. So, take deep breathes and remember that you have done your best before the test.

2. Once in the exam room, read the instructions, take your time. You will be handed a cardboard and markers to write on. To start your test in a calm manner, write a powerful positive quote at the top right corner. This is something I learned while in nursing school

from my maternity professor. Any form of positive affirmation is good.

3. I always start my exams by writing down the priority concepts. All of them. This is just me. This habit has helped me maintain a certain amount of focus every single time and I stand by it.

4. Begin the test. Read the questions in entirety. An answer will pop up in your head after you read the question. Look for the objective closest to what your initial thought was. Choose the answer and keep going.

5. Once you select an answer. Click next. Do not read the question again or change your answers. Keep it going.

6. If you are to spend more time on a question, let it be time reading and re-reading the question to understand what it is asking before you answer or read the options. NEVER read and re-read answer options because every time, you will generate a different understanding from the original presented option.

7. Take a break and breathe when you feel overstimulated. Let that oxygen into your blood and up into your brain cells. Then get back at it.

8. When you finish the exam, no matter what your cut off is, do something fun. My friend planned a trip to Miami to avoid focusing on when the results would come in.

If you fail on your first attempt, re-evaluate, and try again. Like the detour I mentioned earlier in this chapter, things happen. It is not the end of the world even though it might feel like it is.

I know great nurses that have taken the NCLEX twice, thrice, and even five times. You must be honest with yourself. Whatever did not work in the beginning, do not continue to do. You might need refresher courses on topics that continue to challenge you or review priority setting. Whatever you do, do not give up. Remember, once you are a nurse, no one will ask you how many times it took to pass the exam. Passing the exam is all that matters.

Take a break and get back to it. You are not a failure and you are not a loser. You just did not test well at first. It is not the end of the world if you fail the NCLEX the first time around. Below is advice from two nurse friends of mine who had to retake the exam.

Stephanie Rosario, BSN, RN

1. How many times did you retake the NCLEX?

I took the NCLEX 3 times.

2. How long did you wait before you had retake the exam?

When I failed the first time, I waited about six months before I tested again, due to being discouraged and having little time off from work to study. When I failed for the second time, I waited about four months until I retook the test.

3. Did you change your review methods? If so, what did you do differently?

When I studied for the NCLEX the first time I focused more on reading content and trying to memorize what I was reading. I did not spend much time working on practice problems. When I studied the second time around, I still focused on reading content, but also incorporated a lot more practice problems. The final time I studied, all I did was practice problems. I did not touch any of my content books. I did practice problems on my own and with my nurse friends. What I found the most helpful about doing practice problems was reading the rationales of why an answer was right, but also reading the rationales as to why an answer was wrong.

4. What tools did you use for review?

The last time studying I used an app called UWorld. This app was by far the best studying material! It thoroughly went through all the rationales for each answer. It also allowed me to make my own tests, either general or content specific. The first two times studying I used content books from nursing school, and general content based NCLEX study guides I bought.

5. What advice would you give a student that has to retake the exam?

The advice I would give to a student nurse that failed on their attempt is to never give up, no matter how many times it takes! Push through and believe in yourself. You made it through all the hard, trying times in nursing school. You will make it through this test! Do not obsess over memorizing content. That is what nursing school was for. Focus your time on answering practice problems. Really dig deep into the rationales and understand the why is and how is of an answer, do not just memorize the answer. If you understand the rationale as to why an answer is wrong or right, then you can apply that knowledge and understanding to other questions as well. You got this!

Kelly, BSN RN

1. How many times did you take the NCLEX?

Twice

2. How long did you wait before you retook the test?

I took it the first time in the first week of August and then I took it again late September; you must wait 45 days at least to retake the exam.

3. Did you change the way you reviewed the second time around? If so, what did you do differently?

Yes, I did more book work as opposed to online quizzes and tests. I just went through the Kaplan NCLEX book from front to back and reviewed that way with everything I needed a refresher on.

4. What materials did you use?

Kaplan NCLEX book.

Notes from classes in the past

5. What advice would you give to a student nurse that failed on their first attempt?

I would tell them they know themselves better than anyone. They know how they learn. I was told to do online work and to do the ATI books, but that is not how I learn. I must go through everything and write everything down. I work better with pen and paper than on a computer. And I would also tell them to relax. It is just a test, and you can take it again. Each test is different, and it does not prove how good of a nurse you are or are not. Also, if you fail at 75 questions it does not mean you are stupid. I failed at 75 questions and the second time I passed at 75 questions. It does not represent how good I am as a nurse.

Post NCLEX

After soaking up the fact that I had passed and added initials to my last time. I started to plan yet again.

An incredibly wise instructor of mine from Regis College said, "When nurses advance in practice, two critical aspects deteriorate. These aspects are: communication and assessment." This is what happens. We should become more polished in these areas with more advanced education and not less. This statement encouraged me to be a better practitioner should I chose to advance my education. After NCLEX, we secure a job. If you can, take a vacation or break before this process. If you must then let us talk about how you can secure a job.

CHAPTER 12

Job Hunt and Securing a Job

―――――o―――――

Job Hunt

THE FIRST TIME IS ALWAYS EXCITING. YOU MUST CHOOSE YOUR FIRST NURSING JOB WISELY; IT MIGHT JUST SHAPE YOUR WHOLE NURSING CAREER

As new nurses, our minds are fresh and we, like sponges, absorb everything. In my opinion, it would be ideal for employers to hire new nurses into new specialties because unlike old nurses whose ways you have to change, a nurse that is entirely new to the profession is equivalent to a brand new car with no mileage—whatever you put on accumulates and you can only build up from there. New nurses are also like blank slates.

Before I graduated, I made sure to ask my professors to write my letters of recommendation. I had my eye on a nurses' resident program at my place of work. I also figured that by the time I took the exam, the instructors would be off from school or on vacation. Then it would be much harder to reach them. I had already chosen my area of interest and made sure to ask professors that have at least worked in these areas to write my recommendation because they would speak to the need for me to work in that area, understanding my capabilities.

We have always been told that your clinical placements are job interviews per say.

After having tried and failed to get into the hospital as a PCA. I applied to the same floor I had my first clinical and I was hired. I made sure to network and create connections that would place me in the areas where I needed to be. Networking is crucial for a nursing student. You never who you are going to need.

The people we network with will not only be resources, they will be colleagues and even friends. I have been told that nursing is a small word. Therefore, working in a hospital environment is beneficial. Even if you do not get into that same hospital, you will always have an open door in the future and a reference or two. My first nursing instructor and work supervisor wrote my recommendation letter for a nurse residency at another hospital.

After my practicum, I drafted an email to the unit manager and expressed interest in working on the floor. The floor where I had my practicum is a cardiac intensive care floor. I was discouraged from pursuing a position on this floor because I was told, "They do not usually hire new graduates." I pursued the position anyway.

While working on the same floor, I had crossed paths with two new graduates that were hired and extensively trained through a nurse residency program. They seemed competent and I said to myself, I do not care what I am told, I will proceed with the application process, if they do not hire me, another hospital will.

Two weeks after graduation, I updated my resume, I emailed my professors and made them aware of the fact that I would be requesting references as soon as I get licensed. I also sent in applications to all floors I was interested in with the note "pending NCLEX certification." Too early? I would say not. At the time, I wanted to work as soon as I was licensed.

With many of us are vying for positions in the hospital, being ahead of the bunch will not hurt you but motivate you. This is especially true if you are looking to start within a nurse residency program.

This process works very well for a student that is planning to work immediately after nursing school or as soon as they take the board exam. Many of my nursing colleagues started working within two months of being licensed. Others took time off, enjoyed their families and travelled the world with plans of returning to work later in the year.

How soon you start working after leaving school has nothing to do with how good of a nurse you will be. We are so competitive as student nurses we forget that we have earned an education. No matter when or where you go, how soon you practice or in what specialty., it all does not matter. What matters is what kind of nurse you will be when you start to practice. Do not be pressured. Your calling will come to you. You will find your niche.

I know someone that had to take the board exam several times before passing. This individual I could tell was going to be a great nurse. All she had to do was beat the test. She was what you would call an angel. Very diligent, kind, patient and understanding, she possessed all the worldly qualities of a great nurse. She finally passed the exam on her fifth try and is indeed a great nurse now.

What we should be doing is our absolute best and everything else will fall into place.

Coloring Outside the Lines

I wanted to be a critical care nurse for so many reasons, many of which I have relayed in this book. I heard the negatives. People told me that newer nurses rarely got into this field. The most ridiculous negativity I heard was that I will not be hired because of the color of my skin. By observation, few nurses of color are not hired into critical care fields. This one I laughed off at first, but it is the reality, and something should be done about this.

I know my capabilities. I speak of this to assure you that confidence in yourself is much more important than what other people say. Without the former, the latter will be lacking. Someday I will be hired into a critical care field and I will certainly encourage other nurses of color to pursue fields they are interested in.

One day as I was dragging through my day, a potential interview asset crossed my mind. See, during my practicum, we were assigned to author a paper on the ten competencies of nursing. We were to use our clinical experience and find examples within the facility we practiced and use them to reflect on the knowledge, skills and attitude a new nurse should have to transition into practice.

I wrote and researched the ten competencies well and planned to add the paper to my portfolio. I wanted to let the interviewee know that I was a well-rounded student, and more than skills, I was ready and eager to learn about the organization I work with. My plan was to print this paper out and leave it behind after I had interviewed or simply place it in my portfolio. Add your stellar nursing school papers to your portfolio.

I also knew that I had given my all in every one of my classes and clinical rotations. This meant that no matter where I went, I would be a good nurse. Yes, you have an interest, but you could also color outside the lines. Go into a field you never expected, learn, become skilled and then move on to your field of choice armed with more experience.

Securing an Interview

As I have mentioned on multiple occasions, I had my practicum in the cardiothoracic intensive unit. Having worked at the hospital for close to two years, I knew my way around the human resource department and the department head for the unit I was interested in. I emailed the department and made calls to the human resources department.

I also was applying to other area hospitals and called them frequently to inquire about the status of my application. I knew of people that had jobs within a month of earning their licensure and those that had no work for a certain period. Finding a nursing job is individual based. Do not grow weary when you do not have an offer. Continue to search.

The idea of having clinical experiences in multiple fields is to find what you love and what speaks to you as a person. Most seasoned nurses recommend that starting out as a medical surgical nurse makes you a well-rounded nurse. My interest was critical care. I put a lot of emphasis in getting into a specialty in the beginning of my job search. I only wanted to apply to critical care units. One could argue that it was too soon for a specialty, but I can affirm that with the proper education and training, new nurses can be successful in these fields.

Many new nurses say that they will take any job as long as it pays the bills. Some students are more worried about their student loans and other expenses and would rather take the first offer than work a little harder at what they want. Not to blame them, but this is the way this country is set up. We are constantly gravitating towards the next thing with little to no thought because we are afraid that we will miss a chance, an opportunity, a bill. Yet the truth is, there is a place where you belong but if you go too quickly somewhere else, you might miss what is really made for you.

This could be a contributing factor to new nurse's low retention rates. Nursing is beautiful, but you must belong where you go. If you do not, you might find that nursing is not what you hoped it would be. You are not where you should be. Like a puzzle piece, you must take time to find your niche for you thrive and belong.

Preparing for the Interview

Here is the realty, you will send out over 50 applications, change your resume to match different hospitals and follow through with multiple human resources departments. Searching for your first job after nursing school is an errand.

After multiple emails and calls. I managed to secure an interview for the unit I was interested in. I really had no idea how to prepare for the interview. I usually have gone to interviews unprepared and just interviewed well but this was different. This is a professional interview for my first nursing job. I wondered what they were looking for. The only thing I was a hundred percent familiar with is the unit and what I had learned there.

I always have been resourceful. I thought about my resources. What was within my reach that would ensure that I nailed this interview? I am a part of a social group of black nurses that have been incredibly supportive and offered great counsel on several occasions, so, I thought, why not reach out and gather advice from a variety of people? I wrote a post on their web page inquiring about first time interviews and what to expect.

There will be times when you have no idea how things will go, then you would have to ask someone that has lived the experience to guide you. Therefore, a nursing network is valuable be it in employment, education or even lifestyle. We all need each other.

As new nurses, we need guidance such as "what to expect during and post nursing school." Nursing schools have done an excellent job preparing us academically but not enough in some areas. For example; how to prepare and secure your first job or how to interview for success in your initial interview.

For many, a nursing interview is a first. My first interview was with a nurse residency program at a hospital I had worked for close to two years. Attaining a job in a novice nurse program was important to me. Novice nurse programs smooth out some of the loose ends and prepare new nurses to take on a professional role using a faculty model guidance like nursing school. Also, the easiest way to get into a specialty is through a nurse residency program.

How to locate nurse residency programs

- Research area hospitals and find out when these programs commence, how many student nurses are taken, and what the requirements and commitments are. You might consider visiting the HR departments at these hospitals. Know the requirements ahead of time and collect required material. These programs have strict deadlines. You need to have all the information ready.

- Join Indeed.com and create a profile and search for new graduates' nurse residency programs. You will receive notifications everyday indicating what residencies are open.
- Attend nurse hiring fairs in your community.
- During clinical rotation, make sure to ask your clinical instructors whether their hospital will be hiring in a new graduate program. Also request references from your clinical faculty ahead of time. Valuable information to have is their email and phone numbers as well as the units they work on.

These programs are highly competitive. The requirements included should be available for an application to be considered and accepted.

Requirements for residency programs;

- Recommendation letters from instructors, nurse leaders and work places
- Essays stating your interest in the organization and why you went into to nursing
- Proof of GPA, diploma, and nurse licensure

- BLS certification
- Prior experience especially if you are applying for an area of specialty
- An updated nursing resume
- References (emails and phone numbers)

Above are the general requirements, make sure you have everything they request to place yourself at an advantage.

Things to do to make your resume stand out:

- Are you looking to get into pediatrics? Take the PALS. Stand out from the rest of the applicants.
- Take the ACLS course and update your BLS.
- Are you looking to stand out while applying to a cardiology unit? Take refresher Telemetry courses and attain certification
- Join nursing organizations in your area and become an active member.
- Add all your leadership and sportsmanship achievements to your resume.
- Do you belong to any honor societies? Make sure to add them as well.

The Interview

I interviewed for three residency programs. The first residency program interview was at Tufts Medical Center for an intensive care unit, then Mayo Clinic in Florida for cardiology med-surg and lastly, Boston Medical Center for a medical surgical position.

The first time for anything is always a gamble. At Tufts Medical Center, I interviewed with four nurses. At Mayo Clinic in Florida I interviewed with human resources and then I had an online interview with the unit nurse manager. The toughest interview was Boston Medical Center where I had a round table interview with nine nurse managers.

How to prepare for nursing interviews

- Prepare a portfolio. In this portfolio, include your stellar work from nursing, leadership, sportsmanship, volunteer work at various organizations, your diploma, nurse licensure, all other licensures that apply to nursing (current BLS, ACLS if you have one), and at least four resumes for the team. Remember to create an index for your portfolios so the interviewer knows where to find the information they need.

- Research the organization extensively. Become familiar with the mission statement, hospital background, what makes the institution stand out and its uniqueness. How do you relate to the organization and its mission? Nursing is a profession of relationships. We should build a working relationship with the organization to succeed. Researching the organization will help you figure out whether you want to be affiliated with the organization. Your values should mirror those of your place of work.

- Research the units you intend to work on. What cases are they taking? What is the patient population? What is a nurse on the unit expected to do? This will structure your answers to address the population you seek to care for.

- You are now a nurse. Assess yourself extensively. What are your weaknesses and strengths? For every weakness, list ways you have improved on them in the past. Interviewers are not looking for a perfect candidate; they want to see honesty and a genuine sense of willingness to learn.

- Pick a professional outfit. Something comfortable that makes your presence felt and memorable. I would go with a suit color that is memorable. Make sure to wear your hair and make-up in a professional manner as well.

- For Tufts and Mayo clinic interviews, I was the least prepared. These interviews were a month apart and I never researched the core of the interviews. Having worked at Tufts, I assumed I knew the core values. I also was noticeably confident. I focused on my skill set for both interviews because both residencies were not specific about what the requirements were at the time.

- Boston Medical Center however clearly stated that their nurse residency was based on the ten competencies. The ten competencies include professionalism, team work and collaboration, leadership, systems-based practice, information and technology, evidence-based practice, quality improvement, patient centered care and communication. For each of the competencies, you should have an example from the clinical setting. State how you applied the competency, what skills and knowledge did you attain, and what was the attitude you demonstrated that made you successful and teachable.

- Practice nursing interview questions with a colleague—a colleague preferably in health care profession to focus the questions and critique your answers.

- Prepare questions to ask at the end of the interview. Do not ask about pay or how soon you can take a vacation.

- Remain open to shifts and always state that you are available to start with the stated start date.

- If possible, find out how many people you will be interviewing with. That way you are not shocked when you walk into a room of ten people like I did.

- Review your resume. Your resume should have only nursing related work experiences. Be noticeably clear and concise when you state the duties completed as you will be asked to review these during your interview. There should be no errors. Have someone proofread your resume if possible.

- Inform your references that you are looking for work. Have them give you the dates and times they are available for calls and emails should attempts be made to reach them become futile. Place your references in your portfolio.

- Use your network. If you know nurses, talk to them about the interview.

- Lastly, change your resume to match the job requirements they are searching for so that you are highly compatible. This places you ahead of others.

Interview Day

- Arrive an hour early for the interview. I was ill prepared for my first nursing interview. I honestly just winged the interview. Arrive early and practice your relaxation techniques. The more prepared you are for an interview, the calmer you will be.

- Introduce yourself, pay attention, and write down who is participating in the interview. You will be emailing each one of them, thanking them for the opportunity to interview.

- Hand a copy of your resume to everyone in the room and keep one for yourself. That is your guide. Practice what is on your resume so you can speak about the contents without reading directly from paper.

- Pace yourself. Do not feel pressured to answer immediately. Take a minute and then answer the question.

- When answering nursing interview questions, answer them using the SBAR communication tool. For every question where you are told to give an example, state the situation, your role, give a little background, and talk about how you perceived and responded to the situation and then add what you could have done better. Clearly state how you learned from the situation, how your attitude was influenced and what skills and knowledge you attained. Organize all your responses in this manner. This is how nurses communicate. Learn to casually use this tool in conversation.

- When the question you are asked is clinical in nature, follow the nursing process (assess, diagnosis, plan, implement and evaluate) and use your priorities when asked about two critical patients. If the interviewee presents an emergency, your initial response should be to call for help and start resuscitation measures. If the situation is not an emergency, assess and then state how you would act. They are trying to assess your ability to think and act like a nurse. Nurses prioritize and apply critical thinking.

- Know the ethical guidelines and when presented with an ethical dilemma, answer the question with an ethical principle it applies to.

- Know the institute's mission statement, apply the mission statement, and share how you relate to it when asked why you want to work at the institution. Why you chose a work place is based on your values compared to the organization you intend to work with.

- Do not speak of future goals that involve returning to school within a year. This is not the time or place. You are new to nursing and your focus is on acquiring skills. These places are more concerned with commitment because it takes a lot of money to train new employees. This does not mean that you be without future goals. Just do not mention them yet.

- Never sell yourself short. This is the one time you should not. Do not be afraid to tell them why you are the best woman/man for the job. I called myself boring because I am all about work. I know. You totally rolled your eyes at this. I have no idea where that came from. The things we say when we are nervous are shocking sometimes. I sold myself short. Do not. I repeat, do not ever sell yourself short. Not in nursing, not in life. And of course, I am extremely far from boring. At the time, that answer sounded perfect.

The other mistake I made was to shun interviews from areas that I was not interested in at first. I was called about an operating room nursing position and I simply said I have no interest. Every interview you score, you should go to. The more you interview, the better you get. These multiple interviews will also prepare you to succeed when you finally find the position you want.

There is a clinical component to the interviews and as a new nurse, you should be prepared because they are assessing your skills. You are expected to have the skills from the clinical setting. This is the area of the interview I felt I did poorly in. I know my skills, but I was not prepared to speak of them in my interview at Tufts Medical Center. Looking back, I should have been more elaborative.

After the Tufts Interview

I knew I sold myself short at this interview and did not do enough research. A week after the interview, I had not heard back from human resources. I called and left an email requesting an update.

Human resources reached out to me and said that they were still interviewing other candidates. That is never a good sign. If you are what the interviewees want, the search stops and the interview is closed off. I later found out that I was not considered for the position. I was gutted. I felt that I had done everything right. Worked two years at the hospital had excellent grades and from what I knew then, my clinical instructors were impressed with my skills and knowledge.

One of my colleagues was also terribly upset upon hearing that she was not selected. I said to her, "This is not going to take away your education nor the fact that you are nurse. It does not even mean that you are not good enough. It just means that someone fit the description of what they were looking for. You will still practice and sometimes, when things happen to us, we are pushed toward our calling. Fast forward, she is working as an emergency room nurse at a reputable Boston hospital and recently started to travel.

I emailed human resources and thanked them for the opportunity. I also emailed the nurse in charge of the program to let her know that I was interested in other positions should there be any available. The thing with nursing is that it is a small world. We must not burn bridges because who knows who you will need some day. Never underestimate the power of networking. Make sure to leave all relationships open no matter how upset you are.

As soon as I was done with this. I sat down to rethink my way forward. I hoped to get into the cardio-thoracic ICU and that did not happen. My best chance was at this hospital and if luck would have it, another hospital would offer me the position, and that time I was better prepared.

Was I disappointed that I did not get that first position after having worked with the hospital? Absolutely! But what I was grateful for was the experience and the skills I learned that would prepare me for whatever role I would soon practice in as a nurse. I am very hardworking, and, in that moment, I knew that I will one day be in an ICU.

I applied to several other places, emailed my references ahead of time and let them know that I was actively searching, and they should expect calls. I reached out to colleagues working at other hospitals, asked if the floors they worked on where hiring and asked that they put in a good word for me.

A nursing colleague of mine went as far as asking if she could hand my resume to her floor manager to place me in a better position to be hired. Knowing someone always puts you a step further.

Frustration will kick in when you see statements such as "no newly graduated nurses," on job positions but do not lose faith. Remember, you have the education. There are individuals that have had no work for at least six months after graduation, but they never gave up. Keep searching.

Finding a new job as a new RN is tedious. It almost feels like a full-time job with no pay. Changing those resumes and cover letters to match every organization requires organization.

I created a checklist to make sure I was following up on every one of my applications.

Job Checklist

Organization	Cover Letter	Updated resume	Follow up application	Interview date	Follow up interview
Hospital #1	Sent	updated	completed	12/10/18 Portfolio ready	
Hospital #2					
Hospital #3					
Hospital #4					
Hospital #5					

***If you need to add details about the interview, you can enlarge your interview box to include details. Having at least four portfolios ready will save you time when you are called to interview. I used binders from Staples to compile my portfolios.

Following up on the Tufts Medical Center Interview

I wrote a letter to the chief nursing officer requesting a meeting to better understand why my commitment to the hospital and good academic standing did not get me a position in the RN residency program. Within a week of sending the email, I was able to meet with her and we had a fruitful discussion. I was upset but I needed to know the details so I could better my chances of securing a job in other institutions.

She had carefully investigated my situation and in my understanding, in comparison with other competitors, my commitment was lacking. See working at this hospital, I made a mistake and chose work requirements that were extremely challenging to meet during nursing school. I was working per diem one day a week. I also had a full-time home care job at the time.

Being per diem a week meant that I had to commit to one day a week. Something that proved to be a challenge in school as I was also working at another job. Because this book is focused on highlighting my mistakes, achievements, and shortcomings in hopes that future nursing students would do better, I recommend per diem work when you have enough wiggle room. Always choose per diem monthly positions. I requested to change to a monthly per diem, but my request was not met because of staffing issues. The manager said I would have to quit something I was not able to do at the time. I was learning on the job and hoped to work at this hospital upon graduation. So quitting was not an option.

Nursing school is a challenge. You will have weeks that are more challenging than others. During this time, the focus should be on school. Should your schedule open (that is, during times where you are not testing), you will be able to pick up work. Knowing your schedule and being on top of it is crucial to avoiding inconsistencies. The ideal situation would be not to work at all. But remember, working in a hospital or health-related facility will sharpen your thinking.

While meeting with the chief nursing officer, we also agreed that there should be rubric and/or guidelines to reiterate the selection process for the RN residency programs especially for internal applicants and nursing students that have had placements at these facilities. Guidelines such as what is required for one to be able to compete for a position in the residency program. I think guidelines such as these will enable students to remain accountable while vying for extremely competitive positions.

We also talked about increasing diversity in the hospital's nursing work force. This was a concern of mine and continues to be. I am debating whether I should dedicate my life's work to this cause.

The CNO recommended that I meet with one of her staff who would help prepare me better for interviews because I personally felt that, that was my weakness to begin with. The meeting also yielded inquiries into whether nursing programs prepared their students for interviews and such.

The following day, I wrote to the career placement officer at my former school to inquire about the need to prepare student nurses for professional nursing interviews because as you will find, these interviews are different from what you are accustomed to.

Student nurses' organizations and the nursing faculty can benefit from organizing mock interviews before graduation to equip students with these skills. Career development can also aide in these transitions.

You will also find that searching for work at the end of the year as opposed to the beginning is a challenge as well. A staffing agent informed me about the end of year budgets in hospitals and other organizations. Organizations have fiscal year plans, by year end, the funds have been exhausted. This makes job search at the end of the year more challenging because many organizations have exhausted their hiring budgets.

My job search and nursing connections enabled me to meet with the CNO of South Shore at the time. Even though he did not offer me a position, he gave me so much insight about securing a professional role.

I did not get into the Tufts residency program. Having done a lot of research, I applied the concepts as stated above and secured a professional role at Boston Medical Center. I was able to secure a position out of over 200 applicants with no connections at the hospital. I did not know anyone working at the hospital. I graduated May 2017, was licensed August 2017 but I never worked in a hospital until May 2018. I also interviewed at Mayo clinic in Florida and had my very first Web interview with a floor nurse manager. While waiting for a hospital job, I scored a position in rehabilitation nursing.

In the following chapter, I explore my experiences in rehabilitation nursing and then at an acute care hospital. I have been told that experience in nursing, no matter the field you go into, adds up and before you know it, you are a well-rounded nurse. While you wait, search for your ideal position, and explore positions that enrich your resume.

CHAPTER 13

Rehabilitation Nursing and Acute Care Residency

Rehabilitation Nursing

Never in a million years did I think I would end up in this type of nursing, but here I was. I had no prior rehabilitation nursing experience. I never had a clinical rotation at a rehabilitation. Having started in rehabilitation, I think nursing schools should I consider having students at these sites for exposure.

My initial plan was to start with rehabilitation and move on because nursing is nursing no matter where you are working. Working in rehabilitation cemented my understanding of continuing care from acute care settings to rehabilitation and then back into the community. A critical care nurse focuses on reviving life to a functional level (stabilize). A med-surg nurse manages acute conditions therein and restores functional level. If the level of function is not attained in acute settings, patients are transferred to rehabilitation. A rehabilitation nurse strengthens functional level and foresees discharge into the community once functional level is attained, and a community health

217

nurse then manages conditions within the community. No matter where we practice as nurses, we are a part of a cycle that stabilizes, restores, maintains, and sustains health. All nursing levels are equally important; failure on one level affects the other.

Rehabilitation nursing is one of the least appreciated yet the most challenging types of nursing. Nurses are overworked and underpaid. The nurse-patient ratios are also unrealistic. Some rehabilitations have a 1: 22+ ratio. Ideally, these are supposed to be very stable patients. This is not the case because with the elimination of Long-term Acute Care rehabilitation centers (LTACs), sicker patients are being sent from acute settings to rehabilitation centers. Rehabilitation nursing is med-surg nursing on steroids—the patients are sicker, and the ratios are even higher. I have so much respect and appreciation for rehabilitation nurses. The work they have to do with the resources available to them is outrageous.

Rehabilitation Nursing is Med-Surg Nursing on Steroids

The nurse to patient ratios pose a safety risk to the patients as well the nurses. I initially complained about everything and made comparisons to acute care settings. The only advantage is that there is continuity of care for the patients/residents who live there (long-term residents). It is also easy to notice a change in health status in this population because you get to know their baseline. After a while, I reset my way of thinking and worked through the difficulties. I stopped complaining, comparing systems, and worked. Here is how I made it through rehabilitation nursing.

How I made it through rehabilitation nursing:

- Listen to the patient. Treat the patient/resident not the illness. The most rewarding thing about rehabilitation nursing is that you will form relationships with some of the patients. I had a patient who was difficult but loved chewing gum. Offering chewing gum would make a significant difference in behavior and compliance with treatments. Learn what makes their day better and if it works, that is, make sure it does not affect their health and incorporate it into their care. The turnover is not as high as in acute care settings; you get to have therapeutic relationships with your residents.

- Prioritize and reprioritize. With the nurse to patient ratios, one must stay on top of priorities. There is also a lot of autonomy in rehabilitation nursing. As a nurse, you decide who needs to be sent out to an acute care hospital, and whose health can be managed in the facility. Let us just say, I was always sending patients out of the facility to avoid delays in treatment. Rehabilitations do not have diagnostic services on site. If one needs a chest x-ray, they would have to wait hours before the diagnostic company can come in.

- Delegation in rehabilitations is also limited because the nurses must perform blood sugar checks and vital signs assessments. Nursing assistants in most rehabilitation centers perform only ADLs, or activities of daily living, which includes eating bathing, getting dressed, and toileting. This should change to decrease the workload on nurses. Certified nurse assistants should be able to perform these activities as they do in acute care settings. The nursing assistants are also overworked as well and have heavy patient workloads. The rehabilitation system is failing both nurses and ancillary stuff.

- Set a nursing diagnosis for each patient/resident based on the highest priority need. Unless there is an acute change in health, this nursing diagnosis focuses the plan of the day for this specific resident. That way, you know what their needs are, and you can meet them throughout your day. Keep in mind that the needs might change. Say a new lab result indicates hyponatremia for a resident whose nursing diagnosis was initially just at risk of aspiration. Your plan is going to change. You will then revise the plan of care to include monitoring for: acute confusion, headaches, fluid restrictions, and initiate fall precautions because the health status has changed. Some long-term residents only have labs on a need basis. It is possible that labs, when taken are critical because they are not frequently monitored.

- Save your report forms from the day before. You will hopefully be scheduled to work at least three days in a row. Make note of who has had labs and review the labs at the start of the shift alongside other pertinent information. One of the most important labs in this patient population was testing INR or blood clotting for residents on Warfarin. Keep an eye on the labs, know when the INRs are drawn, dose and dose changes, monitor for bleeding, reinstate bleeding precautions, pay attention to medication interactions, and avoid errors as this would gravely impact health. For example, patients on antibiotics would need to have their INRs monitored more frequently.

- Follow your gut feeling. My strongest skill to date is not ignoring my gut feelings. If something feels off, it is off. The least you could do is follow through and find that it is nothing as opposed to not doing so. Follow and trust your nursing instinct, if it does not feel right, it is not.

- NEVER transfer responsibility because you remain accountable. Just because someone said they will do something does not mean they will. Follow through to the end. I had an experience where a resident/patient continued a medication that was supposed to discontinued. When you receive an order, acknowledge it, and make the necessary changes there and then. This is not the type of information you simply pass on in a report. The oncoming nurse will prioritize based on their own nursing assessment or simply forget.

- Document like your life depends on it. The truth is that it does. Documentation will save you when everything else fails. Remember, if you did not document, you did not do it. With the high nurse-patient ratios, document as you go. In rehabilitation nursing, there is what we call skilled patients. These patients are supposed to receive skilled nursing depending on their admitting diagnosis. These are the patients who need focused assessments and shift notes every single shift. Document the focused assessments as soon as they are completed.

- Compassion fatigue is more likely to occur sooner than later in this area of nursing given the nurse to patient ratio and the nurse assistant to patient ratios. The expectations remain high despite the patient load. The nursing assistants are also working with heavier (morbidly obese and dependent for all care) patients given the high ratio of debilitation from strokes, chronic illnesses, accidents and so on. There needs to be public policy or reform to review staffing ratios in rehabilitation centers. Therefore, nurses no matter the area of practice should be involved in policy. People that are not informed of the patient acuity should not decide what the ratios are. It is dangerous and unsafe for both the patients and the nurses.

- Be open to learning and receiving knowledge. Your attitude about the latest information is what is going to draw the line between a successful nurse and one that is not. The Nurse of Future competences formed by the Department of Higher Education produced 10 competencies that enable a student nurse to successfully transition into a professional nurse. These competencies include knowledge and skills and attitudes a nurse should have to become competent in all these areas. Take initiative and educate oneself, consult facility nurse educators, pair up with experienced colleagues and practice the skills. See one, do one. Most importantly, have an attitude of readiness to learn.

These are a few of the things I learned while working in rehabilitation nursing. The most important take homes in this experience were priority setting and wound assessments. There is a lot of learning involved in rehabilitation nursing and you get to perform multiple skills repeatedly. Starting in rehabilitation nursing made me a well-rounded nurse.

If your intention is to work in acute care, continue to apply to hospitals while working in the rehab setting. Half of the nurses, I worked with in rehabilitation nursing are now in acute care hospitals and are performing well. Some nurses on the other end love rehab nursing and that is their niche.

Acute Care Nurse Residency

I finally landed a med-surg position at Boston Medical Center in a nurse residency program. I plan to grow from here and continue to learn. Six months into the residency and I am grateful for the structure, support, skills, and knowledge that I have attained thus far.

The nursing residency at BMC was organized in a faculty model format where we reported to faculty to mimic nursing school. Then we were paired with a clinical colleague and lastly a preceptor who worked with you for two months following a competency level set by the hospital.

Policy and Protocols

Every organization is different. You are safely practicing if you are following the policy and procedures of the organization you work for. The first thing you will have to do as a new nurse is know where to find the policies and procedures so you can ALWAYS refer to them when in doubt.

You should also know how to locate protocols for drug administration, elopements, and device use among other things.

There are policies, no matter how many times I had reviewed them prior; I still reviewed if I had perform an intervention. These policies include blood administration, heparin protocol, oncology policies, etc. I then decided to print the heparin and blood protocols and have them on my nursing clip board for reference. Keep in mind that these policies are revised often. Pay attention to your emails and organization bulletins to know what the changes are. The only way you are protected in practice is if you performed your interventions as stated in the organization's policy.

Resources

I honestly think that EVERY nurse should strive to be the most resourceful nurse on the unit. Learn where things are, who to page, what pagers, protocol changes, etc. I made a list of the most important pagers and taped them to my badge. I cannot take credit for that though. I learned from another nurse on my nursing unit. Take your scavenger hunt seriously when orienting to the unit. There is a reason for why you are tasked to locate exits, fire extinguishers, oxygen shut off valves, code carts, etc.

Nursing is a part of an interdisciplinary team. You do not have to be caught figuring out something when you have an expert a page away. I utilized all my resources (psych, nutrition, social work, PT/OT). My workplace recently initiated COPD NP to manage COPD care in patients that frequently presented with exacerbations. I think this idea was genius. A medical-surgical nurse assigned 4-5 patients with varying acuity barely has time to complete a thorough education. Leverage your team members and resources.

As a new nurse, you are only as good as your resources. You will have patients that are critical and require increased monitoring or even another set of experienced eyes to guide your intervention. Reach out to your educators, resource nurses, charge nurses, nurse supervisors, and other experienced nursing colleagues.

While working, I frequently looked up significant labs, rare conditions, toxicity levels and their signs and symptoms, etc. Organizations usually have evidence-based, up-to-date information. Use those searches as opposed to Web searches.

Orders and Nursing Orders

Every facility is different. At the facility I work, aPTT lab draws (for monitoring heparin therapeutic levels) are nursing orders. Learn what orders nurses can and cannot place. Every organization, unit and specialty is different. Never carry out an action simply because you were able to do it elsewhere. Always inquire. Knowing the orders, you as a nurse can implement to drive patient care saves time for everyone.

I also learned to review my orders every four hours over my nursing shift to make sure I had implemented everything assigned to me during the shift. It took me one time of missing an order to review how I practiced.

Remain inquisitive. Always question orders that do not apply to your patients. Do not simply implement every order the physician makes. I also have learned that talking about the patients with your colleagues can refocus you. Our nursing views differ, and we can always learn from other professionals. We do have shared goals.

Reviewing Continuously

A nurse that thinks they know it all will soon meet their downfall. A wise nurse once said, "When you are done learning, it is time to leave the profession."

Learning is an ongoing process because new evidence comes up every now and then that changes the way we practice. Know where to locate up-to-date information and always be willing and open to learning no matter how much you think you know. We are in the business of saving lives and if we knew everything, no one would die. There is still so much more out there. Stay open. Your attitude will affect your ability to learn. Change your attitude about acquisition of knowledge, there is a lot to learn out there.

Nurse Bullying

Unfortunately, this vice is a part of both nursing school and the profession. Bullying in nursing takes on different forms. The bullying can be as subtle as assigning heavy assignments to nurses, discounting the care and knowledge level of a black nurse, undermining care, and intimidating new nurses. Travel nurses for example are always "being dumped on." I also have heard newer nurses complaining about the workload because there is a rite of passage that involves working your way into having a say in your assignment ratios.

If one is constantly assigned a workload that is unsafe, as a professional nurse, I would let my charge nurse know that the assignment is "hefty" and if possible, have the assignment reviewed. If this continues, approaching a nursing manager would be the next step.

The bullying or one could call it "nursing while black experiences" I have encountered in my short practice has a lot to do with my accent and skin color. I have consistently had to put my foot down because someone made fun of the way I spoke or simply assumed I was not fit for my role as nurse because I am black. Patients will at times discount your knowledge level as well simply because you look and speak a certain way. I once had a patient send me out of the room to find their nurse because they thought, that a black person was not capable of being their nurse. I am constantly referred to as a nurse's aide (which is fine, I have been a nurse's aide and enjoyed my role).

My approach with colleagues has been to put an end to the bullying by; making the bully understand that what they are doing is unacceptable, unprofessional and will require follow up with management if they continue to partake in the bullying.

When bullied by my patients, I always stop and rethink my next reaction. I do let them know politely that I am indeed educated and licensed to take care of them. I also follow up with stating the plan of care and explaining my role, their diagnosis and building rapport. I have found that in most cases, patients are apologetic.

Patients are the bosses and have a right to make decisions about who is involved in their care. The approach of switching nurses around because a patient requested a nurse that is not black is wrong simply because it creates intolerance.

I also have found that nurses who stood up for one another often had someone return the favor when the need arose. If you notice that someone on your unit is constantly being assigned "multiple critically ill and heavy patients" (those that require multiple tasks and monitoring), make it known that it is unfair and have your peers and charge nurses review their assignments. This creates a culture of togetherness, team work and collaboration. It might not always work but it is a start. Be the type of nurses you expect others to be if roles were reversed.

Holistic Care

Whenever you care for a patient, think creatively, and cover other factors that are contributing to the presenting illness. I had a patient that had 14 admissions within 2 months with the same chief compliant. On further assessment, the team found that the patient was non-compliant and did not take the prescribed medications. When I sat down with the patient, I explored the psychosocial factors contributing to frequent hospital visits. A recurring reason was that the patient needed a place to stay during the winter time. They purposely did not take their respiratory and cardiac medications and ate a lot of salty food so they would then present with both CHF and COPD exacerbation and have a warm place to stay for a week or so. I love working with a safety net hospital for reasons beyond nursing. The populations we serve are unique and most times, there are services we can offer that one cannot find anywhere. I reported my findings to the physician who then assigned a social work consult for the patient to find out what was available.

Nursing care involves the physical, mental, and spiritual aspects of health. I have found that psych evaluations are an essential part of nursing interventions because a lot of the patients presenting to acute settings lack the coping skills to deal with new and past diagnosis. Mental health is often under looked yet the impact on healing and/or health is detrimental. Practice an all-encompassing approach and request as many consults as necessary to care for your patients.

Navigating your Computer System

Knowing how to EFFECTIVELY use your computer system will save you a lot of time and make you more efficient. Remember, time is of the essence. My current workplace uses EPIC health care systems. EPIC is one of the most popular health care systems. In the beginning, I was overwhelmed with the system but with time became proficient. I used YouTube to learn diverse ways of documenting and learned how to auto populate information. Learning how to use the system will ease your workload. The more you use the system, the better you get. I always ask other nurses how they were able to document, enter information, and I keep learning about the system. If you have an opportunity to learn how to do things differently, take it. There are nurses that learn only the basics and become comfortable. Do not be that nurse.

If you are still challenged consult with your IT team and team mates that are well versed with technology.

Working 12-Hour Shifts and Holidays

Some students have not worked through school and are not familiar with nursing schedules and holiday commitments. Working for a facility during school will come as an advantage because you will be familiar with nursing schedules. The adjustment will not be as tough. The most challenging is working on holidays. Over time, you will get accustomed to this requirement.

Working Night Shifts

Nights are the best shifts to learn as a new nurse. The pace allows new nurses to build their own nursing knowledge, allows ample time to perform skills and navigate systems without pressure from management. If this is going to be your first-time working nights, you are going to need help. I have worked nights for about six years. Its challenging. It was hard to get used to them. Here are a few tricks:

- Make sure to ask your colleagues how they have managed to adjust to these shifts. People have all sorts of advice. Listen and try everything until you find what works. Nights can easily take a toll on your life and health if you do not make the right adjustments. I found that my body cannot handle more than two nights in row. I stay away from three nights in a row.
- Drink lots of water during your shift.
- Eat less carbohydrates during your shift. I rarely eat during night shifts.
- Avoid eating after 12 am.
- Stay active. Walk and talk to peers if you are not too busy.
- Work out before the shift and take a shower.
- Do not schedule too many nights in a row until you are used to nights.
- I have heard people use melatonin and other sleep aides, but I would personally advise against them because after a while, they are not as effective. There are foods that are high in melatonin. You can consume them once you get off your shift; foods such as, bananas, rice, ginger, etc., will help regulate your sleep patterns.
- Do not drink coffee past 3 am so you can sleep when you get off the shift.

- Stay up late the night prior to work shift to adjust your internal clock.
- Stay up until 12 pm and go to bed at 12 pm the day of shift.
- Everyone in my circle knows I work nights. I do not take calls or answer messages when I go to sleep. Minimize destructions when you sleep. One of my aunts has a huge sign posted outside her house that says, "I work nights, do not ring the doorbell or call my phone."

Scheduling

Unfortunately, as a new nurse, you will not have much control over the scheduling in hospitals because of seniority. When choosing holidays off, vacations, etc., seniority takes effect. You will quickly become accustomed to this and you will soon move up the ladder yourself. If you have not worked in a hospital setting, this will be quite challenging but like everything in life, you will make it work.

Some nursing positions do not have the weekend requirement. You will be extremely lucky if you settle in positions like these. In the beginning, however, you will have to settle.

Utilize applications such as a nurse grid to stay ahead of your scheduling. If you work in a setting that allows you to self-schedule, set a phone reminder to sign up so you have an opportunity to dictate when you can and cannot work.

When your colleagues ask for shift exchanges, actively try to help them out if it is feasible. You never know when you are going to need someone to cover your shift.

In this chapter, I only introduced you to the basics of my acute care residency. In the following chapter I delve deeper into the lessons I learned during my residency and summarize my first year in nursing. Should you have an opportunity to start with a residency program, take it. It is worth the while.

CHAPTER 14

First Year in Nursing Practice: Lessons

Lessons from my First Year in Nursing Practice

Authoring this book has been an incredible coping mechanism for me because it helped me refocus my thoughts and deal with the disappointments I experienced along the way. I speak of the times that I did not meet the mark of an excellent nurse, the times I did and what I learned.

Every one of the times I fell short, I devised new ways to alter the outcomes and avoid repeating near misses and mistakes. I will at times speak of other observed incidences that are not my own in hopes that the nurse that you become is cautious. You are walking into A LOT! The things you experience, hear and witness will at most, shock you. At the end of the day, what matters is what you learned, and what skills and knowledge you acquired.

The Nurse of the Future (NOF) competencies developed by Massachusetts Department of Higher Education and QSEN competencies that are created for nursing and graduate programs all use Knowledge, Skills, Attitude (KSA) as an indicator that learning has occurred.

Without knowing, I subconsciously used these competencies to amalgamate learning. Here is a few lessons from first year of nursing. These lessons include the knowledge, skills, and attitudes I acquired as I improved my approach to caring for patients. Learning however is an ongoing process, and I will still be learning twenty years from now.

Lesson 1

Two days after receiving recognition for doing an excellent job, I missed a telemetry order for one of my patients. I was devastated. I kept going back and forth about what could have gone wrong during the time my patient was without telemetry. My patient had a very recent CVA history and that was the reason for the telemetry order. My preceptor did not reprimand me; she encouraged me to devise means in the future that would prevent this from happening again. This of course did not help me feel better. I had had a long day with my patients and was honestly trying to stay afloat and remain positive.

The nurse that was taking the report from me is the one that caught the mishap. She had arrived early and had reviewed the current orders prior to taking a report from the previous nurse. This is a practice I have now adopted. As new nurses, the amount of information we are presented with is enormous and these times are truly challenging times for most of us. Devising a personalized checklist became my next focus. Now I review my orders every four hours and before I acknowledge orders in EPIC, I make sure to review all the orders and ONLY acknowledge orders after I have completed them.

In the beginning, arrive at least 30 minutes early and go through your assignment. Look at chief complaints, including PMH (Past Medical History) that relates to admitting diagnosis, current orders, and medications; read admitting MD notes and previous nurses' notes to have the most current events; review last lab values and tests, and note last vital signs. I even personalized my EPIC screen to include last vital signs.

Receive reports and meet patients. During bed safety hand offs, flush IV if there are no continuous infusions. The worst thing would be a change in a patient's status and the IV is not functioning. This happened once. A patient had a potassium level of 6.0 and had lost IV access while she slept.

Prioritize. Compare medications due and note what medications are time sensitive and which ones are not. Insulin and IV antibiotics are often the priority. However, things might be different on the floors you are assigned to.

Knowledge: Connect patient diagnosis with pertinent labs, tests, and interventions.

Skills: Personalize EPIC screen to include vital information, review orders at the start of every shift and every four hours, review patient chart prior to shift start, and create shift checklist.

Attitude: We are human, and we make errors. As nurses, our errors must be minimized to almost none. Seek new ways of performing care, recognize the errors I made, and find creative ways to avoid repeating the same mistakes.

Lesson 2

One day, I was assigned a patient on CIWA scale with no orders for benzodiazepines should they score. The patient had up until then received PRN benzodiazepines every time they scored. The CIWA protocol has a benzodiazepine sliding scale but sometimes MDs order CIWA monitoring without the sliding scale. I noted that the patient had no coverage and had not scored for at least 8 or so hours. I thought there was no urgency to request a sliding scale. WRONG! As a safe nurse, I should have anticipated the needs of the patient and paged the covering MD to add coverage ahead of time.

When MDs order medication, the pharmacy verifies the medication before you can pull it from the Pyxis. This process I learned that day can be long. Fast forward to 6 hours into my shift, my patient scores. I page the covering doctor who then orders the medication, but it took the pharmacy up to one half hour to verify the medication. This experience itself taught me to review medications prior to the start of the shift and most importantly to ALWAYS ANTICIPATE PATIENT NEEDS.

Knowledge: Anticipate needs ahead of time and become familiar with order sets specific to diagnosis, equipment, etc.

Skills: Review medication orders. With time, you will become familiar with order sets. For example, an oncology patient might require PRNs for pain (pain management), nausea and vomiting, etc., even though they deny pain or nausea at the time. Always have the PRNs ordered, verified and available for when you need them.

Attitude: I developed a "better safe than sorry" attitude. I would rather have orders in place and not implement them than to not have orders at all and delay patient care.

Lesson 3

Every nurse will occasionally have an assignment that is busy. I had an assignment where all my patients had a lot going on. One of patients' blood sugar was below 30 and another patient's aPTT was greater than 180 on heparin drip. I also had a confused manic patient and a total care requiring frequent checks and positioning. The latter would have been manageable had we not been short staffed that day. I paged the MD, notified the charge and resource nurse, and focused on the patient with hypoglycemia after stopping the heparin drip for the other patient. The same patient with hypoglycemia was in respiratory distress and not responding to interventions.

I had a lot of help and other nurses were hands on inquiring whether there was anything I needed help with. One thing I know about myself is that it is hard for me to pass on responsibility. Asking another nurse to medicate my patient because I am caught up with another has always been challenging. Other patients however will need to have their needs met regardless of what is going on with another.

Prioritizing your assignment at the beginning of the shift is not the problem, re-prioritizing your assignment because priorities have changed is the problem. I would set a pace and think, okay, now I am good only to have my whole plan thrown off. As a new nurse, wanting to do the most for your patient is the norm. How to let go and let others help is also a challenge because then you will feel useless and so incompetent. Where is the balance? How does one let go?

I found that being a med-surg nurse requires more than one's ability to prioritize. It requires constantly thinking on your toes and having a seamless ability to multitask and apply both the art and science of nursing to save one's time.

Knowledge: Set priorities and re-prioritize, maximizing all your resources

Skills: Delegate as much as possible, relying on teamwork and collaboration, and maximizing resources. The patient that required frequent positioning would be delegated to the nursing assistant. Your role is to make sure this task has been completed as delegated.

Attitude: I appreciated the value of team members, saying thank you a lot more.

Lesson 4

Delegating!! Boy oh boy! No one listens to the new nurse. Delegating in nursing means that a nurse can pass on tasks to another member of team but maintains accountability. Nurses usually delegate to nursing assistants and other nurses. There are five rights of delegation (right task, right circumstance, right person, right communication, and right supervision) and unless you meet all the rights, you have failed to delegate appropriately.

I have been a nurse assistant myself and I could swear I was one of the best. Always thinking ahead, asking my assigned nurse what is going on and just working together with the nurse. I just did my best. As a new nurse, I found that most of the older nursing assistants are set in their ways and that they need to warm up to you first before they take direction from you. Some will assume that because you are a new nurse, you have no idea what you are doing.

Many times, the nurses are younger and are intimidated by the age difference. This can lead to failure to delegate appropriately and in the end, nurses feel overwhelmed with duties.

I once worked with a nursing assistant that constantly disregarded my direction and went ahead to perform tasks as "they always have." I had to set the pace and correct this behavior before it was too late. I pulled the nursing assistant and made it known that what she was doing was wrong and that it affected the delivery of patient care. I went on to caution her against continuing to disregard my direction. I made it known that should the behavior continue; I would involve both my charge nurse and the unit manager.

I am glad the nursing assistant took it well and we have since had a great working relationship.

Knowledge: Delegate and learn the five rights and accountability.

Skills: Develop clear and concise communication centered on respect.

Attitude: I understood that I remain accountable for delegated tasks.

Lesson 5

Keep the team updated. Report any and everything that concerns you and make suggestions. Using the Situation, Background, Assessment and Recommendation (SBAR) concept, I will introduce this patient scenario and the lessons learned from this specific scenario.

Situation: My patient's K dropped to 2.7. Team notified. Received new orders to replete potassium.

Background: 70-year-old male from the Dominican Republic, presented with a small bowel obstruction. Now on NGT to low wall suction (explains the loss of potassium) to decompress bowel. No significant cardiac history

Assessment: Monitor for hypokalemia signs and symptoms, NGT output, focused GI assessment, cardiac and musculoskeletal assessments (Think systems affected by Potassium loss and prevent harm)

Recommendation: Requested that patient was placed on telemetry. Low or high potassium irritates the heart muscle and causes arrhythmias. I wanted to be able to assess cardiac status. Most times, providers have low concern to place patients without a cardiac history on telemetry. I always say no significant history does not equate to no history.

Always listen to your nurse instincts. Even though you will understand that the potassium dropped because of the continuous suction, preventing further harm is a key area of focus. When you are uncomfortable, mention that to the team as well. Turns out the patient needed telemetry.

You will learn that certain groups of patients do not have primary care and will present with chronic illnesses that have not been managed overtime. No significant history does not always mean no history. Just like you will learn that No Known Allergies in a patient that rarely seeks medical care is a reason to be concerned. You will be watching every drug you introduce because you do not know this patient.

Knowledge: Safety, Risk reduction and team work and collaboration

Skills: Effective communication with team to attain the best patient outcomes. Focused assessments of systems you predict changes in

Attitude: As a new nurse, you will at first struggle with patient advocacy. It takes time. Remain open learning new ways to communicate effectively. Observe how experienced nurses communicate. You will learn in time. Nurse instincts are a real thing. Follow your nursing instinct.

Lesson 6

Try to build a good relationship with everyone. Units are known to have their fair share of drama. Avoid that. No one likes a messy person. I personally love to know something about every nurse I work with, so I can relate to them better. Things like how many children they have, or the last place they went to vacation. Little pieces of information like these are conversation points. Oh, and never assume, ALWAYS ask. I learned this the other day after I assumed my colleagues' children were their grandchildren. Oops! Always ask.

Knowledge: Team work and collaboration

Skills: Using effective and respective communication techniques Building cohesive teams that work well to maximize patient care outcomes

Attitude: Respect differences and restrain from making unfounded judgements about your co-workers

Lesson 7

I admitted a patient from the emergency department that presented with SOB. The patient had a restrictive lung disease. Upon reaching the floor, the patient's saturation was 88%. I was told in a report that the patient lived at 85% and was well above their normal. I did not worry. VBGs were did not look great (7.32/77, resp. acidosis), but this case, it was a chronic problem, so I did not put it at the top of my priority list. One thing I should have done sooner was place the patient on continuous oxygen monitoring to keep an eye on their levels while they slept. If you think it, do it. I thought about placing the patient on continuous monitoring but did not follow through. There is a reason these thoughts cross your mind. Nursing instinct!

Fast forward, an hour or so later, during routine vital signs, my patient saturation drops to 70% on 4 liters of oxygen. After reassessing and checking my equipment, I panicked. I placed the patient on non-rebreather and called in more help from the team. The patient was placed on an oxymizer and then a CPAP machine.

If you think it, act on it. Always assume what could go wrong and stay ahead of the illness. Think, what is the worst thing that could happen? Then prepare in case it does. Now, naturally, when I am assigned a patient with SOB, I request continuous oxygen monitoring, especially if their saturations are low. I want to see what happens when they fall asleep. I review the last VBGs; I set up the room with a tank, non-rebreather.

This same night, I had a sickle cell disease patient with a hematocrit of 12.5 and a hemoglobin of 4. The patient refused to sign consent for blood, and I was keeping an eye out for that patient as well. Nevertheless, I made sure my type and screen was current and was prepared should anything go wrong. My other patients needed IV antibiotics around the clock. This was the type of night were my prioritization was on steroids. I was constantly re-prioritizing and barely took a break. At the end of the shift, one of my patients gave me a tight hug and suddenly, my whole night meant something. Despite the night I had, I was not as tired anymore. Nursing is so rewarding!

Knowledge: Apply evidence-based practice and use equipment to monitor patient.

Skills: Anticipate patient needs, prepare for emergencies, and set priorities.

Attitudes: I recognized that I could have done better, and I learned from past experiences how to practice better in the future.

Trust your nursing instinct. If you think something is wrong, it is.

Lesson 8

I had a patient on continuous fluids for hydration. My patient had one peripheral IV. I went into the room to give an IVP and forgot to reconnect the fluids. I realized at the end of the shift while passing on report to an oncoming nurse.

At this point, I knew had to review my checklists to never miss this important task again. I created a new way to complete takes for all my 4-5 assigned patients. When you fail, revert to the basics. Now my check lists are in the ABCs format.

ABCs

Airway and breathing: Is the patient breathing on their own? Do they have supplemental oxygen? If yes, what is the saturation on the supplement. Oxygen is medication, do they have an order? What is their respiratory history? Do they have chronic illnesses in exacerbation? Do they use CPAP/BiPAP? What respiratory medications are they on? Are they currently SOB? Will they need a bed-side commode to alleviate decreased work of breathing? What do their ABGs look like? What is their cardiac function? My unit transitioned to a hematology/oncology unit, which means I was now being assigned patients with compromised airways (trached).

Questions and assessments included the rate of humidified oxygen, saturation, suction orders, extra trach, etc.

Circulation: Is this a cardio-pulmonary patient? What is their cardio-pulmonary history? Is this a renal patient? Are they fluid overload or deficit? What is their blood pressure? Are they on any fluids? What fluids have they received in the past shift? Are they taking blood pressure medications? What medications are they taking? Are they on telemetry? What is the rhythm? Have they had any changes? Do they have IV access? Is it patent? Lab results related to fluid volume (Na, K, BNP...)

So far, my priority self-checklist is working. I am also reviewing my orders in the work-list at the beginning of the shift and every four hours to make sure I did not miss anything. Therefore, arriving before time is so important.

Knowledge: Information pertinent to patient diagnosis

Skills: Utilizing checklists to complete complex tasks

Attitude: Recognizing that you need to improve previously learned information and being open to new ways of doing things.

ABC Checklist

Airway	Breathing	Circulation
PMH: Lung disorders, acute respiratory conditions,	PMH Lung disorders, acute respiratory illnesses, spinal cord injuries above C6, ENT cancers	PMH: cardiopulmonary, cardiac, renal disorders
Presentation	Presentation	Presentation
Equipment Trach? Supplementary Oxygen?	Equipment Trach? CPAP? BiPAP? Emergency equipment	Equipment EKG
Interventions Saturation? Meds? Neb tx? PRNs	Interventions Acute vs chronic management? Saturation? Humidification? Suction? Anti-anxiety meds? PRN nebs? ABGs/ VBGs?	Interventions Telemetry Peripheral IV access IVF? Fluid restriction? Dialysis? Weights? Outputs? Electrolytes BNP? Diagnostic tests? (stress tests, Last Echocardiogram ...?)

*** You can personalize these checklists to mirror the floors you work on.

Go back to the basics, that is foundation thinking when you are lost. Your foundation in nursing is what will ALWAYS hold you up.

Lesson 9

I forgot to draw labs on one of my oncology patients. While going about my duties, I saw one of the older nurses print the lab labels, place the labels and tubes in a bag and taped the bag to the door in the room as reminder. Older nurses are gold mines! I have done this since I observed this nurse and now, I have not forgotten to draw labs since.

Medical surgical units are terribly busy, and you will be performing so many tasks at the same time. Learn new ways of recalling information or create a personal checklist to help you recall. Checklists are an absolute necessity. I have also developed a personal checklist for oncology patients.

Personalized Oncology Patient Checklist

Cancer type	Mets? Focused assessments of affected symptoms
Chemo?	Last chemo, type of chemo
CBC	Think safety Replacing everything as along as it is needed
Chemo side effects	Mucositis, n/v/d
Port access	Blood return, all labs changed to unit collect, s/sx of infection at site,
Vital signs	TEMP***
Pain management	Meds? Effective?

***This type of checklist will only work if you are in a specialty unit. It is impossible to have checklists for all medical-surgical conditions. You can formulate checklists based on systems to clue you in on what the most important tasks are.

My medical unit recently merged with hematology and oncology and there is a lot to learn. Consulting with peers and reviewing hospital policy as well as evidence-based practice is important to stay afloat and practice safely. Your seasoned nurses are gold. I am learning a lot with this new population and forming a checklist has been a great tool so far. A colleague just taught me how to calculate the absolute neutrophil count the other day.

Knowledge: Specialties require one to build a knowledge base in the said niche. Refer to evidence-based practice to navigate specialties.

Skills: Utilizing checklists, observing experienced peers, and asking questions. Consult with educators assigned to your floors. Obtain certification in areas where you are lacking.

Attitudes: Learning in nursing is a continued process. We are always learning. Maintain an open attitude towards new information. Never lose your inquisitiveness.

If I were to list every single one of the lessons, I have learned in nursing in the first year, I would have a 500-page book for you. Learning is never ending. I will continue learning throughout my career. Every day I come in to work, I learn something new.

There is always a new condition, anomaly, unique way of achieving positive outcomes. As a novice nurse, your role is to learn. Soak in everything. Let the ones before you pour into you. Take your lessons and learn from them. Do better and be better.

I have attached two interviews from nursing colleagues about their first year in nursing. I hope that these first-year nursing experiences can enlighten you as well.

Interview with Diane Zatolokin, RN

1. What area of nursing did you start your career?

I started my nursing career in a Level III Trauma Emergency Department (ER).

2. Tell us a little about your specialty and how you settled into your professional role in the first year.

The Emergency Department is a fast-paced specialty with a quick turn-around rate no matter what time of day. Working in any Emergency Department is overwhelming and tiring, but exceptionally exhilarating. I work with medical/behavioral adult and pediatric patients. An ER is notorious for having 2-5 hour wait times. The nurse patient ratio is typically 1:4-5. The highest patient amount I had was 6 patients at one point!

During nursing school, I always wanted to start in the ER or an Intensive Care Unit. Starting off as a new graduate nurse in the ER, I was beyond nervous and was judged for the first six months of my career. When older nurses found out I was a new nurse in the ER, they immediately questioned me and asked why I did not start on a medical-surgical floor to gain some experience. I would just say, "I got lucky with this job." You must try your best not to feed into the work drama. My preceptor who trained me for six months is one of the smartest and hard-working nurses I know. I was fortunate to feel comfortable with her and she was so patient with me. If I become half the nurse she is, I will be so proud of myself!

After reaching the six-month mark, I was officially on my own. The first two months being off orientation was difficult. I felt nauseous going to work every day. I felt incompetent and my anxiety was highly increased. My scheduled hours a week were only 24 hours, but I forced myself to work 40 hours a week, which I still do. I do this because it forces me to be more comfortable with the ER experience and procedures. Once you get comfortable with adults, the charge nurse will send you off to the pediatrics ER. Here, the anxiety and feeling incompetent starts up again! There were shifts where I felt myself becoming overwhelmed and I had to go to the closest bathroom because I would cry my eyes out for 1 minute and then get my emotions back together because you have to go back on the floor to take care of your patients. When you spend more time with the pediatric community, the more comfortable you will get. I hated working in pediatrics not because of children, but because of how hard it is. For example, when you place and intravenous (IV) in an adult, it takes one nurse. When you place an IV in a child especially from newborn age to school-age, it takes two nurses, one nurse assistant, a child-life specialist and do not forget, the parents are at the bedside watching your every move. Of course, not every IV is a perfect placement, certain parents lose trust in you and you become the enemy. Also, with a newborn to a toddler, we, the nurses at times must perform a straight-catheterization for a clean urine sample. Yes, pediatrics is hard.

3. Do you think starting a career in this specialty is worth the while?

Even though starting off in the ER is intimidating, I would highly say it is worth the while. Personally, I cannot see myself working on a medical-surgical floor or any other unit. You start on a blank slate with your patients and you must be the detective with them. From this, you are exposed to some of the wildest patient conditions! For instance: a stroke, myocardial ischemia, pulmonary embolism, respiratory distress, cardiac arrest, flash-pulmonary edema, conscious sedation, shattered femurs on patients who are on blood thinners, E.coli eating away someone's stomach and causing their vitals to be closely unresponsive, insulin and vasopressor drips, and the list continues, etc.

The ER is fantastic place for those who love adrenaline.

4. What advice would you give a newly licensed nurse given your first-year experience?

The biggest advice I would give to a newly licensed nurse working in any unit is, give yourself time to learn and be easy on yourself. You are doing the best that you can. Experience and skills come with time. If you do not believe in yourself, no one else will. Do not let other nurses take your dignity away. You will have days that you love your job and you will have the ones where you hate it and ask, "Why am I doing this?" That is ok! From this, perform self-care tasks and find your go-to nurse resources who are willing to help you. If you feel like you are drowning with your assignments, ASK FOR HELP! Do not put your patient or yourself in danger. Ask someone if you are unsure about a medicine dosage or a physician's order. Experienced nurses love new nurses who ask for help or just ask questions because it tells them that you are serious about your job and that you genuinely want to learn. One of the best compliments I have ever received from a nurse was, "You are like a sponge; you absorb all the information we tell you."

Another piece of advice I will give is, do not act like you know everything because in reality you do not. We learn so much in nursing school but when you go to the workforce, things are entirely different. Also, avoid the work drama! These nurses will turn on you quickly if you complain or say something that you should not be.

One year later, things do get easier but do not let your guard down. Healthcare is always changing and new experiences in your career will evolve, always.

Diana is now a travel ED nurse.

Interview with Mikayla Murphy, RN

1. What area in nursing did you start your career?

I started on a med-surg telemetry floor

2. Tell us a little about your specialty and how you settled into your professional role in the first year.

About a couple of months ago I started at my dream job in labor and delivery. I help with laboring, pushing, delivering, and patients recovering from both vaginal and C-section deliveries. Currently I am still on orientation but will be off in a couple of weeks. LDR is a whole different world and it was much different than what I was used to in med-surg. It has been a transition, but I am so happy I made the move! I dreamt of doing this job since senior year of college, and I feel so lucky to deliver new life into this world each shift.

3. Do you think starting a career in this specialty is worth the while?

I fell in love with labor and delivery during my maternity clinical and I knew it was something I wanted to do. I wanted to get a foundation in, and when jobs opened and I felt like it was time, I made the move. This specialty is amazing, and I am honored to be involved in this type of care. It has been worth the wait and I can see myself making a career of this!

4. What advice would you give a newly licensed nurse given your first-year experience?

The advice I would give to a newly licensed nurse is to ask a ton of questions and to never give up. Real life nursing is nothing like nursing school. It is a transition for sure. Balancing an assignment, prioritizing, critically thinking, talking to doctors, and constantly assessing can be overwhelming for any experienced nurse. Now as a new graduate? That is even harder. It can be intimating, but if you remember why you started, it will all come together. Eventually you find your groove and one day if you are lucky, you get to do exactly what you dreamt of.

The Knowledge, Skills and Attitude (KSA) I used to assess whether I had met my learning needs is a tool developed by QSEN. I personally think that the most important part of this tool is the ATTITUDE. Once you change your attitude, you are teachable and are more willing to learn. The saying "your attitude can make or break you" is true for nursing as well. Be it excelling school or job searches, your attitude can dramatically change the result.

Before we even graduate nursing school or prior to nursing, we have a specialty in mind. I started off thinking that I will be a great pediatrics nurse. In my senior year, I was set on going into critical care. A year or so into the profession, I have not practiced as a critical care nurse yet. Where you practice, what kind of nurse you will become is all a puzzle. Nursing school only introduces us to a fraction of what is available to you. The following section explores this subject further.

What Type of Nurse Will You Be?

A seasoned nurse once said to me, "Which one was your favorite clinical? Your favorite clinical is usually your best fit or nursing niche." Another seasoned nurse said: "I have done about everything, psych, geriatrics, intensive care, etc., you name it. Just keep going until you find what you love."

Most times, we take the first job we are offered, learn, and then move on in search of our true calling God forbid there is a vacancy and you are need of a job to make ends meet. That is how nurses end up in fields they have absolutely no interest in. Of course, with time, they learn to cope. Some fall in love with these new fields while others do not. The latter then spends the rest of their work life miserable, hating their jobs and nursing in general. Some even end up leaving the profession prematurely.

Nursing Types

There are so many types of nursing outside of those you were prepared for in school. Most schools will prepare you for med-surg areas, pediatrics, maternity, acute/critical care, and research and community health nursing for BSN nurses. There is however a wider scope of nursing. There are case managers, clinical liaisons, corrections, travel, infusion nurses, informatics, public health, forensics, nurse researchers, school systems, hospice, etc. This is what makes this field is so exciting. The places you will go, and the lives you will touch are all unlimited.

I cannot stress the importance of a good fit enough. I started out in rehabilitation nursing, and I am now in acute care on the hematology/oncology medical-surgical floor, but my passion is cardiac, and I will be on an intensive cardiac unit soon. I do get a fair number of cardiac patients on my unit and it is always a delight to care for this patient population. I recently learned so much about amyloid and how it affects the heart. I would say this medical surgical experience has given me so much exposure and laid a great foundation. I do think new nurses benefit from starting on medical surgical units.

If you fail to get into your first choice. Take a position that is closest to where you want to be. Sometimes you will find that you fall in love with what you start with and end up staying. For a nurse that wants to end up elsewhere, remain intentional. Make friends in the areas of nursing you want to get into. Find a mentor and someone who can continually remind you of the goals you set for yourself.

My favorite clinical was my nursing practicum in the cardio-thoracic intensive care unit. I remember being told by someone that my chances of being hired on this unit were slim to none. This evaluation had nothing to do with my capabilities but had a lot to do with the black to white nurse ratio on this floor.

To quote this person, "How many black nurses have you seen there?" she asked. There was only one black nurse on that unit. This has never deterred me from pursuing this dream and I have told everyone I know that I will get into the ICU sooner rather than later and I will work on increasing diversity and inclusion in high acuity areas and draw more light on incivility in nursing.

If you have already made up your mind about the area of nursing that suits you, do your homework. Find nurses in that field and ask them to tell you what is important for you to know; how to prepare yourself for the role; what background or training you will need and so on and so forth. Find a mentor and follow their journey closely.

Building Professional Nursing Networks

Building a network is crucial. Not only do they place you at an advantage for securing positions, they are a great support system. If you are lucky to know nurses, talk to them about your fears and concerns and find out if they had similar experiences when starting out. It is also helpful to know how they navigated the system and what helped them settle in.

I got my first nursing job through a connection with a fellow nurse. This lady, God bless her heart, went beyond to secure this job opportunity for me. I sent her my resume, and she handed it over to her boss and then checked weekly with the hiring manager to make sure that I was going to be hired.

Networking keeps you afloat in the profession and it will enable you to meet various successful nurses in the field who might become colleagues or sources of inspiration. Many times, we fall off or lose interest in the things that we love. Having a network of people doing the same work will strengthen your belief in the profession and renew your drive when you sit and talk through your experiences with people doing the same work.

Join nurse organizations that mirror your beliefs and stay active in the communities you reside in. There also many nursing groups on social media that help you stay on top of skills and introduce new research as well as refuel your intentions.

Networks also enrich nurses' lives. Some networks organize activities outside of work that develop the mind, body, and soul. This nurse-time allows for nurses to build relationships while making substantial connections.

In the process of authoring this book, I made several connections with nurses in managerial positions, work, and all fields. I made sure to collect business cards and send thank you emails whenever they allowed for a meeting. Again, you never know when you might need these people again or them you. You have heard the phrase that "nursing is a small world." There is a chance that you will meet these people again.

Everything in your first year of nursing is unpredictable. After beating the NCLEX, securing a job will feel like a full-time job. Like myself, you will have a lot of interviews. Using the rubric, guide, and materials I shared, I believe that it will be easier for you to secure a job.

The next task will be relearning how to practice because nursing school does not teach you everything and yes, practice is quite different from what you learn in school.

Having an attitude of willingness to learn will ease the burden of learning. Do not beat yourself down about the slight mistakes you make in your first year. Learn from your experiences and build up on your nursing knowledge. You will get more confident and yes, you will interact with ease after a while. It all takes time. Pat yourself on the back for having made it this far. Look back at the beginning and see where you are now, a lot will happen, and you will change so many lives. The best is yet to come. Stay put. Welcome to a great profession.

References

Accreditation Commission for Education in Nursing (ACEN) (2018). *Accreditation Manual.*

Retrieved from http://www.acenursing.net/manuals/GeneralInformation_August 2017.pdf

Accreditation Commission for Education in Nursing (ACEN) (2013). *Search ACEN Accredited Nursing Programs.* Retrieved from http://www.acenursing.us/accreditedprograms/programsearch.htm

College Board's College-Level Examination Program (CLEP) (2019) *Key Examination Information* Retrieved from *https://clep.collegeboard.org/about-clep/key-exam-information*

The Massachusetts Nursing Core Competencies (2014). *A Toolkit for Implementation in Education and Practice Setting.* Retrieved from https://www.mass.edu/nahi/documents/Toolkit-First%20Edition-May%202014-r1.pdf

Malvik, C (2019) *A Beginners Guide to Understanding the Levels of Nursing credentials* blog post (2019) Retrieved from https://www.rasmussen.edu/degrees/nursing/blog/different-levels-of-nursing/

National Council of State Boards of Nursing (NCSBN) (2019). *2019 NCLEX Test Plan.* Retrieved from https://www.ncsbn.org/2019_RN_TestPlan-English.htm

Visual Aural Read/Write Kinesthetic (VARK) A Guide to Learning Preferences (2019). *The VARK modalities.* Retrieved from *http://vark-learn.com/introduction-to-vark/the-vark-modalities/*

Epilogue

Y ou can now call me Sandrah Nanziri, BSN RN (more credentials in the future)

Here we are, a year and a half in and still learning. A few years ago, I did not know anything about nursing school. This explains why I titled this book, *From Zero to Nurse.* The book is a lived experience, a personal journey from having no idea what nursing entails to becoming a nurse and then practicing as a nurse. I currently practice as a hematology/oncology nurse and I will return to school for my doctorate but in the meantime, I am focusing on building up on my knowledge and passing it on as I go.

Nursing is such a broad field. You can do a lot with your nursing degree. The nursing process itself has prepared you to approach many life encounters. I utilized parts of the nursing process to start a nursing-based business selling nursing scrub tops in African print. The goal of creating this line was to diversify scrub collections and in turn celebrate the origins of African-American health care professionals. Upon assessment of the current scrub market, I learned that no one was selling professional print scrub tops. I did my research and initiated the Nursey Scrubs in 2018 after years of pondering the idea. Just like everything in life, the beginning is always a challenge. We are however picking up the pace and we will soon be producing prints on a large scale and continue to head in the direction of becoming a global brand that celebrates diversity and inclusivity. To follow this journey, follow @nurseyscrubs on Instagram and subscribe to the website nurseyscrubs.com for frequent updates and deals.

I work full-time and I run a small business. This business is online and most of the purchases have been from face-to-face interactions. I encourage other nurses to continue to pursue other interests. There are nurses running home care health agencies and staffing businesses. They are even sharing their stories on YouTube and becoming authors. The opportunities are endless if you want to pursue entrepreneurship. Without a strong background in English, writing and literature, I have authored and self-published a book. Never limit oneself.

Authoring this book took three years. I hope that the three years I put into this project are worth your while and that I have influenced you to succeed in nursing and beyond.

Made in United States
North Haven, CT
25 March 2025

67229787R00167